The Reality of Nursing Research

Nursing, midwifery and health visiting are relatively young disciplines and are shaped by their location at the interface of academia and practice. As a result, researchers are often unaware of and unprepared for issues which can have a major impact on their work.

Focusing on the nurse researcher's dual role as practitioner and researcher, as well as research ethics and the relationship between practitioner and academic agendas, *The Reality of Nursing Research* helps to:

- locate the practical dilemmas of nursing research in historical and policy context
- prepare those about to embark on research for some of the issues they will face
- reassure researchers that they are not the only ones to encounter the complexity of real life research
- support the research teacher or supervisor in preparing and mentoring their students
- share experiences of others who have encountered similar issues and provide some practical advice on their solution.

This book looks at the real life dilemmas faced by nurse researchers at key stages of the research process from developing a research question through to disseminating the findings. With illustrative case studies and practical advice for nurse researchers it will appeal to teachers of research, research supervisors and nurses undertaking research at diploma through to doctoral level.

Davina Allen is Director of Nursing Research at Cardiff University. She has a background in adult nursing and sociology. Her research interests centre on the social organisation of health care work.

Patricia Lyne was formerly Professor of Nursing Research at Cardiff University. Originally a biochemist, she changed career after being inspired by the care she observed as a volunteer in terminal care. She has since sought to combine the insights of her scientific training with her understanding of health care and health systems to promote research and evidence-based practice in nursing.

The Reality of Nursing Research

Politics, practices and processes

Edited by Davina Allen and
Patricia Lyne

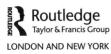

Routledge
Taylor & Francis Group

LONDON AND NEW YORK

First published 2006
by Routledge
2 Park Square, Milton Park, Abingdon, Oxon OX14 4RN

Simultaneously published in the USA and Canada
by Routledge
270 Madison Ave, New York, NY 10016

Routledge is an imprint of the Taylor & Francis Group, an informa business

© 2006 selection and editorial matter, Davina Allen and Patricia Lyne; individual chapters, the contributors

Typeset in Times by
HWA Text and Data Management, Tunbridge Wells
Printed and bound in Great Britain by
MPG Books Ltd, Bodmin

British Library Cataloguing in Publication Data
A catalogue record for this book is available from the British Library

Library of Congress Cataloging-in-Publication Data
A catalog record for this book has been requested

ISBN10: 0-415-34627-4 (hbk)
ISBN10: 0-415-34628-2 (pbk)
ISBN10: 0-203-59705-2 (ebk)

ISBN13: 978-0-415-34627-6 (hbk)
ISBN13: 978-0-415-34628-3 (pbk)
ISBN13: 978-0-203-59705-7 (ebk)

Contents

Contributors

Davina Allen is a Professor and Director of the Nursing, Health and Social Care Research Centre and the Wales Centre for Evidence Based Care, School of Nursing and Midwifery Studies, Cardiff University. She has a background in adult nursing and sociology and has published widely including *The Changing Shape of Nursing Practice* (Routledge 2001), *Nursing and the Division of Labour in Healthcare* (with David Hughes, Palgrave 2002) and the Sociology of Health and Illness Monograph: *The Social Organisation of Health Care Work* (with Alison Pilnick, Sage 2006).

Sue Bale is Associate Director of Nursing at Gwent NHS Trust. She has worked in the field of wound healing since 1982. She has published extensively and frequently presents at international conferences. She is a founder member of the Wound Care Society (1985); the European Wound Management Association (1991); the *Journal of Wound Care* (1992); and the European Pressure Ulcer Advisory Panel (1996). In 2004 Sue received recognition for her services to wound healing when the Royal College of Nursing conferred on her a Fellowship for her outstanding contribution to nursing research, development and practice of wound care in the UK and internationally. Responsibilities of her current post include engendering a research culture within the organization, encouraging participation in research activities, and co-ordinating and overseeing research in the Trust.

Linda Edmunds is Nurse Consultant Cardiac Care, Cardiff and Vale NHS Trust. She has a background in adult cardiac nursing, which has included teaching and clinical roles, with a special interest in chronic disease management and rehabilitation of the cardiac patient and family. She is Chair of the Welsh Cardiac Rehabilitation Group and a member of the Welsh Coronary Heart Disease Professional Advisory Group, and has made presentations at national cardiac rehabilitation conferences. Her role is concerned with ensuring clinical practice is underpinned with research and education and that this is considered as every day clinical practice.

Nicola Evans is a Lecturer in Mental Health Nursing in the School of Nursing and Midwifery Studies, Cardiff University. She has a strong clinical background and a particular interest in therapeutic work with young people. She is a co-opted member of the RCN Children and Young People's Mental Health Forum and represents Cardiff University on the All Wales Children and Adolescent Mental Health Service Senior Nurse Advisory Forum. Nicola is a member of the Editorial Board of *Mental Health Nursing* and regularly peer reviews papers for publication.

Lisa Franklin is a Professional and Practice Development Nurse at the University Hospital of Wales, Cardiff. In 2001 Lisa was seconded part-time from clinical practice to the Nursing, Health and Social Care Research Centre in the School of Nursing and Midwifery Studies, Cardiff University to work on a joint research project on how severe pressure ulcers are cared for in the community. Lisa has developed skills in both quantitative and qualitative methods.

Ben Hannigan is a Senior Lecturer in Mental Health Nursing in the School of Nursing and Midwifery Studies, Cardiff University. His academic interests include the organization and delivery of community mental health care, an area which he is investigating in his ongoing PhD. Ben has published widely in the field of mental health policy and practice, and is editor (with Michael Coffey) of *The Handbook of Community Mental Health Nursing* (Routledge, 2003).

Lesley Lowes is a Research Fellow/Practitioner in Paediatric Diabetes in the School of Nursing and Midwifery Studies, Cardiff University. In her research role she supervises nursing research, co-ordinates a Chronic Childhood Illness research programme and is developing a research agenda in paediatric diabetes. Lesley is a member of the Editorial Board of the *British Journal of Nursing*. She has many published papers relating to both practice and research and is the co-editor (with Ian Hulatt) of *Involving Service Users in Health and Social Care Research* (Routledge, 2005). Her clinical role includes the management of a paediatric diabetes nursing team, holding a case load of children and teenagers with diabetes and undertaking nurse-led clinics.

Patricia Lyne held the RCN Chair in Nursing Research at University Wales College of Medicine until 2002. She is a Non-Executive Director of Conwy and Denbighshire NHS Trust. Her research interests have centred on the provision of evidence-based nursing care, encompassing methodology and evidence appraisal. She has been involved in the development of research policy at local and national level and was formerly a member of the editorial boards of *Journal of Advanced Nursing* and *Clinical Effectiveness in Nursing*.

Chris Martinsen has 15 years' experience as a clinical nurse in Critical Care at the University Hospital of Wales. Chris was seconded part-time to the Nursing Health and Social Care Research Centre, School of Nursing and Midwifery Studies, Cardiff University to work on the design of a model for sustained development, dissemination, implementation and evaluation of local clinical practice guidelines. This involves a multi-disciplinary development group with academic and clinical representatives in order to ensure both scientific validity and clinical applicability. He has presented work at international nursing and medical conferences.

Sally Rees has a background in adult nursing and is a Lecturer at the School of Nursing and Midwifery Studies, Cardiff University. She was awarded a part-time secondment at the Nursing, Health and Social Care Research Centre to contribute to a literature review on changing nursing roles in primary and community care. She has a particular interest in the students' transition from pre-registration to qualification and has undertaken research on the experiences of newly qualified nurses. She has participated in collaborative research with social work lecturers on shared learning between nursing and social work students on qualifying programmes in Wales.

Philip Satherley is a Researcher in the Nursing, Health and Social Care Research Centre, School of Nursing and Midwifery Studies, Cardiff University and Deputy Director of the Wales Centre for Evidence Based Care. He has a background in social science with a substantive focus on systematic reviews, evidence appraisal and qualitative evaluation. His recent work has focused on developing appraisal systems for the research and practice communities, which is reflected in his publications and conference outputs.

Keith Weeks is a Principal Lecturer in the School of Care Sciences, University of Glamorgan. He is a science and education graduate, with an extensive background in adult nursing and science and mathematics education applied to health care. He has undertaken research involving the educational needs of nursing students. Following completion of his PhD he has developed a growing international reputation as a subject specialist in constructivist-based learning and the research, design and construction of 'Authentic World' learning environments. Within the latter context he holds the post of Learning Environment Design and Development Director at Authentic Word Ltd, a spin out company of the University of Glamorgan and Cardiff University.

Foreword

Nursing research may not be the first on your list for bedtime reading but those immersed in practitioner-based research will find this is something of a page-turner! Research in nursing has been dominated by debates about funding and capacity-building. This book signals the change in direction by focusing on the research/practice relationship in its many forms and manifestations. Might this suggest that nursing research has come of age? Certainly the relationship has been a recurrent feature of nursing curricula – and one which sets it apart from other academic disciplines such as medicine. In fact, it would not be an exaggeration to say that the research/practice relationship has been something of an obsession within nursing, one over which the respective communities have agonized at times. However, casting these roles as simple dualities underestimates the complex relationship between the two. A key strength of this book is the refreshing perspective it adopts in critiquing the research/practice relationship, moving beyond cliché to produce a subtle and sophisticated synthesis. This is expressed both in terms of lively case studies in the second part of the book and an adroitly argued analysis in the first. The book takes as its starting point the policy and political drivers which have configured relationships between practitioners and researchers in different ways. It then provides us with an archaeological dig into how those relationships have been shaped by different contexts and settings; academic, professional and relationships with research participants. The unique contribution of the book lies in the experience and expertise its editors bring through their respective academic training in sociology and life sciences. The benefit of this lies in the editors' abilities to weave in their own methodological training and research experience into the analysis and enter the ethnographic world of research in nursing from these standpoints. Case studies are 'home-grown' and add a rich texture to many of the substantive points made in the first half of the book. This is accomplished in a style which is both elegant and accessible. Nursing research has surely come of age!

Anne-Marie Rafferty

Preface

In most disciplines, even those which are long-established, researchers find themselves in uncharted waters when they begin the voyage from an initial research idea. Feeling safely prepared by their experience, education and training, they are surprised by the unexpected complexity of research in the real world, where leviathans such as political expediency and resource limitation, not to mention personal or professional animosities and ambitions, lurk below the surface. Accounts of major scientific discoveries sometimes tell the story of such experiences and hint at these unexpected aspects of research, but they are rarely formally described. Instead they become part of the tacit understandings of a field of knowledge which, in mature disciplines, are absorbed through exposure to the culture of the related community of scholars.

Nursing[1] research is a young discipline and lacks some of these established traditions. Although it shares many of the challenges faced by other fields, it is also shaped in fundamental ways by its location at the interface of academic nursing and clinical practice. This sets nursing apart from pure disciplines such as sociology and life sciences which do not have to deliver a service, but highlights commonalities with other applied fields such as social work, medicine and engineering, which all have to contend with this duality in advancing their knowledge base.

We argue that the voyage of the nurse researcher in addressing the academic and clinical dimensions of their identity and in resolving the political dilemmas encountered in their relatively young discipline will always reveal some particular hazards, challenges and opportunities which are not normally described or considered during research preparation. As a result, nurse researchers are often unaware of, and unprepared for, issues which can have a major impact on the process and outcome of their work. These are rarely addressed directly by research methods texts and, despite the trend towards an increasingly reflexive approach to research, uncut stories of projects rarely make it into the public domain. The aim of this book is to address this gap in the literature. We write from our own, UK perspective, and while important developments have gone on elsewhere, we are not in a position to describe these in the same way. Nonetheless we believe that our observations have wider currency for nurses in other healthcare systems.

We begin in Part I with a critical consideration of the nursing research context. We analyse the characteristics of nursing research as both a knowledge form and as a knowledge community and examine the broader political and policy framework in which it is located. We explore nursing's heterogeneous and segmented character, the divergent social worlds of academe and practice and the wider competing and overlapping discourses which shape the field. This provides the basis for a critical consideration of the apparent consensus within nursing about the place of research in the profession, culminating in Chapter 5, in which we underline the breadth of the nursing function and make the case for a better understanding of the different modes of research engagement across the diversity of nursing roles.

In Part II these issues are considered in relation to specific aspects of research practice. Case study materials are deployed to examine elements of the research process: selecting a topic, negotiating a proposal through key gate-keeping committees, generating data, researching your own organization and/or clients, analyzing data, working in multidisciplinary teams and disseminating findings. It is not our intention to repeat the well-rehearsed insights and debates which can be found in most high quality research texts. Rather, the starting point is the experiences of our contributors, all nurse researchers associated with the Nursing, Health and Social Care Research Centre, Cardiff School of Nursing and Midwifery Studies. Their preparedness to tell their story 'as it really is' has provided us with a unique resource from which to examine the contemporary nursing research endeavour.

We hope that our analysis of the issues nurses encounter in the real world of research will help others to identify and resolve these early in the design of their research and/or be better prepared for them should they arise unexpectedly. As well as providing some practical tools and guidance in dealing with the common problems that can occur, our aim is to contribute to the maturation of the discipline by developing a more sophisticated understanding of issues that all too frequently are considered in terms of the individual research project or researcher rather than the broader political context in which nursing research is undertaken.

Note

1 We use this term to include nursing, midwifery and health visiting.

Acknowledgements

This book has its genesis in a discussion of an issue brought to a research group at the Cardiff School of Nursing and Midwifery Studies which had arisen for one of the group's members at an early stage of their PhD study. We would like to thank Patricia Jones for sharing with us her research experiences which stimulated the thinking on which this book is based.

Abbreviations

BCN	Breast Care Nurse
CFRE	Cardiff Framework of Research Engagement
CNO	Chief Nursing Officer
DN	District Nurse
EBP	Evidence-Based Practice
HEI	Higher Education Institution
NHS	National Health Service
ICT	Information and Communication Technology
MDT	Multidisciplinary Team
R&D	Research and Development
RAE	Research Assessment Exercise
RCN	Royal College of Nursing
REC	Research Ethics Committee
UKCC	United Kingdom Central Council for Nursing, Midwifery and Health Visiting
WORD	Wales Office of Research and Development for Health and Social Care

Part I

The reality of nursing research

Historical and political context

Introduction

In a paper first published in 1994, Jane Robinson discusses her experience of carrying out a research project into perinatal mortality for a UK National Health Service (NHS) health authority (Robinson, 2002). Undertaken in 1981, the research suggested that high levels of local perinatal mortality could not be explained by patient factors, but were possibly attributable to shortcomings in the quality of care provided. The results of the study were angrily resisted by key professional groups, however, and the research report was embargoed. Writing 13 years later, Robinson candidly describes her ambivalent response to these events and the impact it had on the progression of her work.

> On the one hand they encompassed feelings of anger and grief at my powerlessness to be able to use the lessons of the research findings in order to bring about change on behalf of the parents whose babies had died and who had participated so willingly in the research process. Medical power had never seemed so omnipotent as when I realised that despite having uncovered aspects of care which raised questions about the management of some pregnancies, no one was required to consider the implications of the findings for their own professional practice. Paradoxically, on the other hand, I also felt a sense of worthlessness and guilt that I had caused hurt and upset to members of health authority staff (especially medical staff) who, like the parents, had also participated willingly in the research and who had given me access to meetings and to medical records. [...] One of the net results of these ambivalent feelings of impotent anger and guilt was that I found it extraordinarily painful to go back over my data to undertake the analyses of the policy perspectives arising from the study which were needed for the completion of a PhD. For a year I could hardly bring myself to contemplate the work and even then it was only because other people put strong pressure on me and lent me their support that the thesis itself was eventually completed.
>
> (Robinson, 2002, p. 55)

It was only with the passage of time that Robinson was able to reflect upon, and draw out, the social and political lessons to be learnt from her experience. She argues that many nurses entering research are mature professionals who want to address issues which will impact on practice. It is essential, therefore, that researchers are aware that research is a political process and that new knowledge which challenges the status quo will inevitably evoke issues of power and control. She also draws attention to the impact of the identity of the nurse researcher in a medical field and how this subordinate status can influence research conduct. In her case, she argues, it appeared to exonerate those concerned from taking her study seriously and allowed them to attack her findings as inaccurate, whilst ignoring the hard evidence on which they were based. She also concludes that no contract researcher should be left with the 'awesome responsibility' of undertaking the research and coping with the politically infused consequences of the findings and draws attention to the responsibilities of research supervisors in this regard.

The analysis Robinson offers of her experiences of the research process, was undoubtedly facilitated by the fact that she was registered for a PhD in a department of social anthropology, social work and social policy which would have been informed by a world view centred on a critical, socially contextualized approach. We suspect that other nurse researchers faced with similar challenges may mistakenly interpret the problems they encounter as a reflection of their own shortcomings. Robinson, for example, argues that the feelings of guilt she experienced were part of a wider process of subordination in which she, as the bearer of bad news, was made to feel unworthy and mistaken in her conclusions.

This example illustrates clearly that problems perceived to be individual or project-specific, actually have their origins in the broader environment in which nursing research takes place and its associated contradictions, social relationships and nexus of power relationships (see also Seed, 1995). Accordingly, the aim of Part I of this book is to consider this context. It reviews the state and status of nursing research in the UK, examines the historical and political contexts which have influenced its evolution and form and analyses the current culture and how this is shaping the field.

References

Robinson, J. (2002) 'Research for whom: the politics of research and dissemination and application', in A.M. Rafferty and M. Traynor (eds) *Exemplary Research for Nursing and Midwifery*, London: Routledge.
Seed, A. (1995) 'Conducting a longitudinal study: An unsanitised account', *Journal of Advanced Nursing*, 21, 845–82.

Chapter 1

Where are we now?

Davina Allen and Patricia Lyne

Introduction

It is now widely acknowledged that research is every nurse's business and that research evidence should inform policy and practice. Accordingly, in a range of settings throughout the UK, nurses are working to develop the knowledge base for the profession. They are doing so against the backdrop of constant organizational change in both service and educational contexts, change which has generated further uncertainty about the nursing contribution and exerted new demands on people who already have busy roles. Despite this, increasing numbers of nurses have undergone, or are undertaking, postgraduate research training and there has been a proliferation of nursing doctoral programmes. Across health services nursing research strategies have been developed and senior nurses appointed to lead them. The consultant nurse role has also emerged at the pinnacle of the clinical career structure with research as a key function. In the academic context, the most recent assessment of research activity undertaken on behalf of the research funding councils revealed significant progress including: a 20 per cent increase in the number of submissions made to the nursing unit of assessment, an improvement in the proportion of submissions achieving research of international levels of excellence, more staff returned, examples of cross-disciplinary working yielding good results and areas of research strength in national priority areas including: mental health, care of older people, heart disease, palliative care, pain management and maternity care (Bond, 2002).

There is, then, much to celebrate. Indeed the publication of *Exemplary Research for Nursing and Midwifery* in 2002 did just that (Rafferty and Traynor, 2002). Its aim was to 'showcase' examples of excellence in the field. The editors, Anne-Marie Rafferty and Michael Traynor, asked an international panel of opinion-leaders to select examples of research which had been influential either for the profession or for them personally. The result was a 'range of topics, methods and organizational models of research', displaying 'impressive diversity and depth', with each paper accompanied by a commentary about its contribution to theory, method or clinical practice. One of the aims of the collection is to situate contemporary nursing research as part of a longer and broader intellectual tradition. Yet the oldest paper – Menzies' case-study in the functioning of social systems as a defence against anxiety (Menzies, 1960) – was first published in 1960 and although the research is clearly about nursing, Menzies herself was not a nurse. These observations point to a key feature of research in nursing: its relative immaturity as a research-based discipline. In this chapter we examine in more detail the state and status of nursing research in the UK in order to address the question: Where are we now?

Evidence-based health care

Modern health care systems are increasingly informed by a philosophy which emphasizes the importance of basing policy and practice on the best available evidence and nursing has been quick to respond. For some, the trend towards evidence-based practice (EBP) represents an opportunity to advance a wider professionalizing project in which research is seen as providing the foundations for the development of disciplinary knowledge necessary to underpin occupational status claims. For others, its value is rather more immediate. Mindful of the wider health service and economic agenda, research on the effectiveness of nursing interventions becomes an essential weapon in the battle to counter the strain towards skills-dilution and substitution (Tierney, 1993).

The need for an evidence-based UK National Health Service (NHS) was first identified in 1991 with the publication of *Research for Health: A Research and Development Strategy for the NHS* (Department of Health, 1991). The report had its genesis in a House of Lords Select Committee on Science and Technology, which in March 1988 reported on the low morale and inadequate funding of medical research. The strategy aimed 'to ensure that the content and delivery of care in the NHS is based on high quality research relevant to improving the health of the nation'. As the strategy evolved emphasis was placed on information systems (Department of Health, 1993b). The creation of the National Research Register, the UK Cochrane Centre and the York Centre for Reviews and Dissemination in 1993 was followed by the emergence of SIGN (Scottish Intercollegiate Guidelines Network), EPPI-Centre (Evidence for Policy & Practice Information Co-ordinating Centre) and other agencies in order to support the information needs of the service.

In 1998 EBP was boosted further by the introduction of clinical governance into the NHS. In *A First Class Service* (Department of Health, 1998), the policy document which heralded its introduction, clinical governance is described as: 'A framework through which NHS organisations are accountable for continually improving the quality of their services and safeguarding high standards of care by creating an environment in which excellence in clinical care will flourish'. New bodies were created in order to coordinate clinical standard setting. The National Institute for Clinical Excellence (NICE) was established to ensure that authoritative national guidance, based on the 'best relevant evidence of clinical and cost effectiveness' is available for all health professionals on the latest drugs and technologies[1.] National Service Frameworks (NSFs), which addressed the whole system of care, began to be developed to set standards for different patient groups. The Commission for Health Improvement was established to monitor progress and ensure that the highest standards were met, through a rolling programme of 'spot checks'.

The challenges of creating an evidence-based health service are formidable. Clinical governance requires a radical change in health care systems and the behaviour of people who work within them (Flynn, 2002). Critics have pointed to the difficulties clinicians face in utilizing evidence in the context of their daily practice: the lack of time, inadequacy of the information communication technology (ICT) infrastructure and the need for specialist critical appraisal and evidence translation skills. For nursing, however, the issue is rather more fundamental. Even if all the obstacles to the utilization of research in practice could be overcome tomorrow, the brutal truth is that nursing's research base is under-developed, relative to more established disciplines, such as medicine. There are vast areas of nursing practice for which no high quality research evidence exists and nursing's ability to contribute to the health services research and development (R&D) agenda is hamstrung by the small numbers of people who can undertake high quality research (Department of Health, 2000; WAG, 2004).

Nursing research capacity

In most pure academic disciplines, a research career pathway begins with a subject specific degree and progresses through to master's and doctoral level study. The traditional doctorate is widely considered to be the entry qualification of the professional scholar. Having successfully completed a PhD, the neophyte researcher will continue their path to independence, which is recognized to be a long one. In her address to the Smith and Nephew Foundation in November 2003, Lesley Degner (2003) quoted the Executive Director of the National Cancer Institute of Canada as saying that it takes ten years to complete this process and produce an independent investigator. During this period the typical career path will comprise a postdoctoral research post (often on a fixed term contract), a junior lectureship or research fellowship, and promotion through to senior research fellow/lecturer, reader and ultimately a professorial chair.

The research career pathway in nursing is rather different. As we describe in more detail in Chapter 2, pre-registration nurse education is fundamentally a preparation for clinical practice. For the newly qualified nurse, like other applied disciplines such as law and pharmacy, the decision to embark on a research career has to be balanced with the dominant expectation that clinical experience will be obtained. While a small number of local examples of innovative practice exist (Lowes and Taylor, 2003) in the UK there is no clearly established career pathway which enables research and clinical roles to be combined.

For those wishing to develop a research career from a base in practice, routes back into higher education can be difficult. As we shall argue in greater detail later, in many respects clinical practice and academic nursing are distinct social worlds with different requirements. In the absence of opportunities to develop research skills and expertise in clinically-based posts, most new entrants to departments of academic nursing aspiring to a research career will need to acquire a doctorate. Yet the opportunities to do this are limited. Full-time research studentships are rare and postgraduate stipends do not compare favourably with mid-career clinical salaries. Funding streams in the UK are beginning to take into account the singular challenges of developing health services research careers and provide studentships that meet the salary costs of applicants. But with only a very small number of scholarships being supported annually, and with the majority of PhDs being undertaken on a part-time basis, increasing the number of nurse researchers will be a torturously slow progress.

There is, however, some evidence that nursing research is starting to progress. Research by the Centre for Policy in Nursing Research (Traynor and Rafferty, 1998) notes a steady increase in the number of doctorates awarded in nursing in the UK between 1976 and 1993 and although the authors estimated that there were only three hundred nurses with PhDs in the UK in 1997, these numbers are now increasing exponentially, particularly with the development of new style professional doctorate programmes of study (McKenna and Galvin, 2004). Furthermore, a mapping exercise undertaken in 2000 showed that between 1996/7 and 1999/2000 there had been an increase in research-based publications and postgraduate students and more evidence of inter-institutional and international collaboration (Traynor and Rafferty, 2000). Nevertheless, as Traynor and Rafferty (2000) report, despite this growth of research activity, the absolute number of research active staff is still lower than it should be in proportion to other professions.

Aware of the problems experienced in areas of education and research in health and social care, the Strategic Learning and Research Advisory Group (StLaR), a government agency which has a remit to ensure joint working on learning and research issues in health and social care at central government level, has commissioned a project to develop a human resources plan for the educator and researcher workforce. The project team have proposed a joint human resources plan to develop the workforce to support learning and research and have developed exemplar career pathways (StLaR HR Plan Project, 2004). At the time of writing the HR Plan Project resides with the Department of Health and Department of Education and Skills who will be taking the proposals forward. In addition the Royal College of Nursing Research and Development Co-ordinating Centre has been proactive in providing careers advice for those wishing to pursue a career in research (RCN, 2005; Kenkre and Foxcroft, 2001a, 2001b, 2001c, 2001d, 2001e).

Nursing research quality

Since the 1980s UK universities have been required to undergo regular review of the quality of their research activity through a periodic research assessment exercise (RAE). The RAE has existed in many forms over its lifetime, but from 1989 it has been consistently used as a basis for selectively distributing core recurrent research funding. Although the Higher Education Funding Councils of Scotland, England and Wales can, and do, apply different principles for the distribution of RAE funds, overall the 1996 and 2001 RAEs have seen an increasing differentiation of research monies with lowly-rated units receiving no funding.

The RAE entails subject-specific submissions which are assessed by panels representing different 'units of assessment'. Assessment is based on peer review, and increasingly the selective use of metrics (Roberts, 2004). The university decides on which staff to include in its RAE submission, based on the quality of their research outputs over the RAE census period. Evidence is also provided on research income, postgraduate research students, research support, the research environment and the strategic planning process (Bushaway, 2003). Actual funding is calculated on a formula based on the quality of the submission, the numbers of staff returned (volume measure) and the discipline (Delamont and Atkinson, 2004).

In the 1992 RAE more than half the nursing submissions (17 out of 29) failed to produce research recognized as being of a quality of at least national levels of excellence but performance has improved steadily since this time. Indeed the number of departments entering the RAE has increased along with the overall numbers of staff returned (from 397 in 1996 to 575 in 2001) and a higher proportion of submissions achieved research of national levels of excellence (26 out of 43 in 2001) or higher (10 out of 43 in 2001). Notwithstanding these tremendous strides forward, nursing has nevertheless consistently been rated the lowest of all academic disciplines (Lipley, 2002; Robinson et al., 2002).

Nursing research strategy

A recurrent theme in policy analyses, has been the fragmentation, poor coordination and lack of strategic vision for nursing research and its isolation from wider health arena (WAG, 2004; Traynor and Rafferty, 1997). Historically nursing research has been characterized by one-off projects – described as 'shot-gun' (Hinshaw and Heinrich, 1990) research – rather than programmes of activity (Kitson et al., 1997), thus limiting its potential to develop a comprehensive theoretical base (Department of Health, 2000). The underlying reasons for this are complex. One possible explanation is that it is a reflection of the predominance of serendipity rather than strategy in nursing research and the need to respond to available resources (see below). Available funding streams are also heavily influenced by managerial view that research has got to be useful and produce something that can be used immediately in practice, which militates against longer-term projects. Taylor and Cable (2004) suggest that small-scale projects offer research experience to neophyte researchers who might be flattered at being asked to get involved. Such involvement may be important too in establishing local academic-service partnerships. It is also the case that nursing has a relatively small number of researchers faced with a large number of potential research problems. Becher (1989) refers to this as the 'people to problem ratio'. He observes that at a given point in time, in some specialist fields a small number of issues are pursued by a relatively large number of people; whereas at the other end of the scale, there are knowledge areas in which the questions that could be asked are virtually unlimited, but the number of people engaged in addressing them is negligible by comparison. As a relatively new academic discipline, nursing is clearly located at the latter end of this continuum. In nurse education, this is combined with a strong generalist ethos which does not lend itself to the in-depth exploration of an area of interest and a lack of familiarity with the strategies and tactics necessary to building a successful research career to which neophytes in mature disciplines are routinely exposed as part of academic socialization processes.

There are signs that this situation is slowly beginning to change. One clear impact of the RAE on research in higher education has been to encourage a more managed and strategic approach to research activity in order to build up critical mass in discrete research areas. Departments of nursing, like other academic disciplines, have adopted a more programmatic approach as they have gained experience in developing research strategies which maximize RAE performance. In some cases, links between Higher Education Institutions (HEIs) and NHS organizations have become stronger, leading to the production of collaborative research agenda. Nevertheless, it is the case that many research 'strategies' are still shaped to a considerable extent by access to funding opportunities and commissioned research is becoming increasingly focused and specific which can limit the scope to build up new areas and strengths over the longer term (Centre for Policy in Nursing Research et al., 2001; HEFCE, 2001). One of the areas of concern raised by the Nursing Unit of Assessment Panel following the 2001 RAE was that there was almost a complete absence of submissions demonstrating long-term funding for programmatic research and that there was evidence of research foci which would benefit from better coordination and cooperation. The report also draws attention to the vulnerability and fragility of research because of the high level of staff movement between HEIs (Bond, 2002). The loss of a senior researcher can destroy a departmental research theme quite literally overnight.

Within the UK there has been a number of initiatives concerned with the identification of nursing research priorities. Kitson et al. (1997) describe a national priority setting exercise established jointly by the Royal College of Nursing and the Centre for Policy in Nursing Research, as part of a wider agenda aimed at influencing NHS R&D policy in response to the Taskforce Report on the Strategy for Research in Nursing, Midwifery and Health Visiting (Department of Health, 1993a). More recently, Ross et al. (2004) were commissioned by the National Co-ordinating Centre Service Delivery and Organization (NCCSDO) to identify priorities for nursing and midwifery research funding in England. Similar exercises have been undertaken by international nursing organizations such as the International Council of

Nurses (ICN) (International Council of Nurses, 1997). Higher level strategies such as these identify very broad priority areas, such as the nursing workforce and health care outcomes. The challenge for those charged with developing nursing research strategies at a more local level is to identify and clearly articulate specific priorities and to locate their strategy within the complex of political, professional and financial drivers which will determine its direction.

Nursing research funding

There is probably no other major area of public spending in the UK that is based on such a thin research base as nursing, midwifery and health visiting. While investment in research and development in health services generally is notoriously low compared with manufacturing industries and most other service industries, little of that investment is devoted to increasing our knowledge and understanding of the main workforce and the activities they undertake. Nursing consumes 3 per cent of the UK Gross Domestic Product which, with a large publicly funded health system, means that nursing is one of the largest occupational groups as regards government expenditure. Combine this with the realisation that the most crucial issue facing health policy-makers is that of workforce recruitment, retention and skill mix, it is astonishing how little investment has been and continues to be made in research on nursing, midwifery and health visiting.

(Nick Black in the forward to Rafferty and Traynor, 2002, p. ix)

Nursing research in the UK is chronically under-funded. With RAE-linked research funding becoming increasingly selective after the 2001 exercise, most departments in England were left with no core funding to support research activity, despite improvements in overall performance. Moreover, there is no additional dedicated source of funding for nursing research and nurses have limited knowledge of, and access to, research funding opportunities and restricted ability to compete for available funds (WAG, 2004). The outcome of the 2001 RAE showed that much of nursing research was self-funded rather than coming from external sources. In a report produced for the Higher Education Funding Council England and the Department of Health by Task Group 3 (HEFCE, 2001), evidence is marshalled to support the conclusion that that health professions research is under funded in two respects: relative to comparable professions and relative to the size of the professions. Funding is also skewed towards short-term projects and, as we have already noted, there is a shortage of funding for coordinated studies.

In the United States the single most important factor in promoting nursing research has been the National Institute for Nursing Research which was set up within the Institutes for Health. Rafferty et al. (2004) note that the important thing in attaining this achievement was a coherent nursing voice supporting and lobbying for earmarked funding and training. Similarly, in Canada, the Alberta Foundation for Nursing Research (AFNR) was established as a result of energetic lobbying during the late 1970s, at a time when there was unrest in the nursing professions which had escalated to the level of industrial action. In 1978 the Alberta Association of Registered Nurses (AARN) presented the Governor of the state with proposals to develop nursing as a research field as part of the Alberta Heritage Foundation for Medical Research which was to receive a huge endowment. After intensive lobbying and support from the Minister of Advanced Education the Government announced a $1 million fund for nursing research over five years from 1982, creating the AFNR, the first provincial or state programme in the world to be set up exclusively for nursing research. The Board of AFNR turned its attention, very early in its life, to attempts to secure future stable and dedicated funding. In this they were not successful. The Government agreed to a second grant of a minimum of $1 million over the years 1987–92, recognizing the achievements of the first five years. Thereafter government support declined as the economic situation of the state deteriorated. By the end of the second five year term it was apparent that all avenues for permanent funding had been explored and the AFNR continued as a residual body until 1997, when it was officially wound up. However, funding opportunities for nursing research continue through medical and health services funding streams, at both state and national level. The initial support for nursing research produced a cohort of experienced researchers engaged in extensive collaborations with credibility and influence (Alberta Foundation for Nursing Research, 1998).

The success of the AFNR again demonstrates the importance of determined and credible lobbying at a time of opportunity, but its demise reveals the vulnerability of a dedicated funding stream to political and economic changes. It was established by Ministerial order rather than by legislative approval which would have been a longer but more secure process. Reviewing the state of UK nursing research, Rafferty et al. (2004) conclude that there are some grounds for optimism. This positive outlook has its origins in recognition of the changed policy mood in the UK which has witnessed a shift away from a strict multidisciplinary approach, which inevitably favoured established disciplines, to one where it is accepted that there is a need to build capacity in targeted areas in health care. The Department of Health and Higher Education Funding Council for England (HEFCE) have agreed to establish a fund to increase the amount of high-quality research related to nursing and allied health professionals. Resources have been committed to support research capacity building in nursing and allied health professions by The Health Foundation which is investing in England, Scotland, Wales and Northern Ireland. In addition, the Department of Health National Coordinating Centre for Service Delivery and Organization research has seen the establishment of a nursing, midwifery and health visiting research programme which was informed by the priority setting exercise undertaken by Ross et al. (2004) described earlier. The value of a dedicated stream can be seen in the programme established by the Smith and Nephew Foundation which has undoubtedly contributed to research capacity in the field of skin integrity and tissue viability. For example, Dr David Voegeli, a recipient of a Smith and Nephew Foundation postdoctoral award had previously developed skills in laboratory investigation of skin properties (Voegeli et al., 1999). The award enabled him to undertake a programme of work exploring the effect of skin hygiene practices on skin barrier function and skin vulnerability in adults. Subsequently, a midwife (Rapley) was successful in obtaining a Smith and Nephew Foundation doctoral award to work in the team to investigate the same question in neonatal care, with Voegeli as co-supervisor. Thus, the original work formed the basis for progressive development within a skin vulnerability research group.

Conclusions

It is clear from this chapter, then, that nursing research whilst clearly on an upward trajectory, faces many challenges. Most significant are the dearth of experienced researchers able to contribute to the knowledge base for the profession and the limited availability of funds to support research capacity. A paper produced from a workshop hosted by the Chief Nursing Officer (CNO) for England to explore ways of strengthening the nursing and midwifery contribution, (Department of Health, 2000) concluded that lack of professional confidence and co-ordination, as well as institutional barriers (including inadequate funding) have prevented nursing from breaking out of a vicious circle of disadvantage. In this respect, UK nursing research shares commonalities with nursing research in some international arena (see for example, Gething and Leelarthaepin, 2000) but compares less favourably with others such as the USA and Canada. In the next chapter we sketch the history of how it is that we have arrived at this situation.

Note

1   In 2005 NICE was superseded by a new Institute: National Institute for Health and Clinical Excellence. The new Institute was formed following the transfer of the functions of the Health Development Agency to the National Institute for Clinical Excellence.

References

Alberta Foundation for Nursing Research (1998) *Alberta Foundation for Nursing Research 1982–1997: A Time to Grow*, Alberta: Alberta Foundation for Nursing Research.

Becher, T. (1989) *Academic Tribes and Territories: Intellectual Enquiry and the Cultures of Disciplines*, Milton Keynes: Open University Press.

Bond, S. (2002) UOA10 – Nursing. Overall assessment of the sector. London: HERO.

Bushaway, R.W. (2003) *Managing Research*, Maidenhead: Open University Press.

Centre for Policy in Nursing Research, R&D Forum Allied Health Professions, Association of Commonwealth Universities and CHEMS Consulting (2001) *Promoting Research in Nursing, Midwifery, Health Visiting and Allied Health Professions*: Report of the Task Group 3 to HEFCE and the Department of Health. Bristol: Higher Education Funding Council for England.

Degner, L. (2003) *Strategic Development of Programmatic Research in Nursing: What Works and What Doesn't?* London: Smith and Nephew Foundation.

Delamont, S. and Atkinson, P. (2004) *Successful Research Careers: A Practical Guide*, Buckingham: Open University Press.

Department of Health (1991) *Research for Health. A Research and Development Strategy for the NHS*, London: Department of Health.

—— (1993a) *Report of the Taskforce on the Strategy for Research in Nursing, Midwifery and Health Visiting*, London: Department of Health.

—— (1993b) *Research for Health*, London: Department of Health.

—— (1998) *A First Class Service: Quality in the New NHS*, London: Department of Health.

—— (2000) *Towards a Strategy for Nursing Research and Development: Proposals for Action*, London: Department of Health.

Flynn R. (2002) 'Clinical governance and governmentality', *Health, Risk & Society*, 4, 155–72.

Gething, L. and Leelarthaepin, B. (2000) 'Strategies for promoting research participation among nurses employed as academics in the university sector', *Nurse Education Today, 20*, **147–54.**

HEFCE (2001) Research in Nursing and Allied Health Professions: Report of the Task Group 3 to HEFCE and the Department of Health. London: HEFCE.

Hinshaw, A.S. and Heinrich, J. (1990) 'New initiatives in nursing research: a national perspective', in R. Bergman (ed.) *Nursing Research for Nursing Practice: An International Perspective*, London: Chapman & Hall.

International Council of Nurses (1997) *Nursing Research: Building International Research Agenda*. Report of the Expert Committee on Nursing Research, Geneva: ICN.

Kenkre, J. and Foxcroft, D. (2001a) 'Career pathways in research: academic', *Nursing Standard*, 16, 40–4.

—— (2001b) 'Career pathways in research: clinical practice', *Nursing Standard,* 16, 40–3.

—— (2001c) 'Career pathways in research: clinical research', *Nursing Standard,* 16, 41–4.

—— (2001d) 'Career pathways in research: pharmaceutical', *Nursing Standard,* 16, 36–9.

—— (2001e) 'Career pathways in research: support and management', *Nursing Standard,* 16, 33–5.

Kitson A., McMahon, A., Rafferty, A.M. and Scott, L. (1997) 'On developing an agenda to influence policy in health-care research for effective nursing: a description of a national R&D priority setting exercise', *Nursing Times Research,* 2, 323–33.

Lipley, N. (2002) 'Could do better', *Nursing Standard,* 16, 14.

Lowes, L. and Taylor, S. (2003) 'The way forward: would the implementation of clinical research posts increase research capacity in nursing?', RCN International Nursing Conference. Manchester.

McKenna, H. and Galvin, K. (2004) 'Doctoral processes: the scholarly practitioner', in D. Freshwater and V. Bishop (eds) *Nursing Research in Context: Appreciation, Applications and Professional Developments,* Basingstoke: Palgrave Macmillan.

Menzies, I.E.P. (1960) 'A case study in the functioning of social systems as a defence against anxiety', *Human Relations,* 13, 95–121.

Rafferty, A. M. and Traynor, M. (eds) (2002) *Exemplary Nursing Research for Nursing and Midwifery,* London: Routledge.

Rafferty, A.M., Newell, R. and Traynor, M. (2004) 'Research and development: policy and capacity building', in D. Freshwater and V. Bishop (eds) *Nursing Research in Context: Appreciation, Applications and Professional Developments,* Basingstoke: Palgrave Macmillan.

RCN (2005) Research & Development Co-ordinating Centre. RCN.

Roberts, G. (2004) 'RAE is here to stay – and getting better', *Research Fortnight*

Robinson, J., Watson, R. and Webb, C. (2002) 'Editorial: The United Kingdom Research Assessment Exercise (RAE) 2001', *Journal of Advanced Nursing,* 37, 497–8.

Ross, F., Smith, E., Mackenzie, A. and Masterson, A. (2004) 'Identifying research priorities in nursing and midwifery service delivery and organisation: a scoping study', *International Journal of Nursing Studies,* 41, 547–58.

STLAR HR Plan Project (2004) A Proposed Human Resources Plan for Educators and Researchers in Health and Social Care, StLaR HR Plan Project Team.

Taylor, J. and Cable, S. (2004) 'Research in response to local need', *Nurse Researcher,* 11, 56–60.

Tierney, A.J. (1993) 'Challenges for nursing research in an era dominated by health service reform and cost containment', *Clinical Nursing Research,* 2, 382–95.

Traynor, M. and Rafferty, A.M. (1997) *The NHS R&D Context for Nursing Research: A Working Paper,* London: Centre for Policy in Nursing Research, London School of Hygiene and Tropical Medicine.

—— (1998) *Nursing Research and the Higher Education Context: A Second Working Paper,* London: Centre for Policy in Nursing Research, London School of Hygiene and Tropical Medicine.

—— (2000) *Measuring the Outputs of Nursing R&D: A Third Working Paper,* London: Centre for Policy in Nursing Research, London School of Hygiene and Tropical Medicine.

Voegeli, D., Clough, G.F. and Church, M.K. (1999) 'Localisation of microdialysis probes in human skin in vivo', *Journal of Vascular Research,* 36, 334.

WAG (2004) *Realising the Potential: Briefing Paper 6: Achieving the Potential Through Research and Development: A Framework for Realising the Potential Through Research and Development in Wales,* Cardiff: Welsh Assembly Government.

Chapter 2

How did we get there?

Davina Allen and Patricia Lyne

Introduction

Nursing's movement from a more-or-less exclusive base in practice to an academic discipline began only about 40 years ago. It is an example of an 'externally generated discipline' (Becher, 1989); in contrast to those (internally generated) disciplines whose roots lie in the academic realm, it owes its origins to influences outside academia and its genesis, evolution and progression have been intimately bound up with the wider fortunes of the profession.

In the UK nursing's occupational history can be understood in terms of an ongoing struggle between diverse discourses (Traynor, 1999; Dingwall *et al.*, 1988; Rafferty, 1996; Allen, 2001) which has been highly consequential for the development of the profession's cognitive and social structure. The notion of discourse comes from social science and is particularly associated with the work of Michel Foucault. We do not adopt a thorough-going Foucauldian analysis here, but we have found this work helpful in understanding the trajectory of nursing research. Critical for current purposes is the attention that this approach draws to the existence of different ways of thinking about areas of social life. For Foucault, discourses are not simply a way of describing the world; they are a major phenomenon of social power. As a ready-made way of considering a given area of concern, a dominant discourse can preclude alternative framings and preserve the status quo; within a certain discourse there are literally things that cannot be said or thought. Discourses evolve over time in response to wider social, political and economic change. They can also co-exist and reinforce each other or conflict. As well as providing a language and a way of talking and thinking about things, they also encompass a whole range of activities, objects, events, settings and epistemological precepts (Prior, 1989). The discourses pertinent to the evolution of nursing research are those of medicine, professionalism, managerialism and gender. In overlapping and competing ways these discourses have been central in shaping the contours of the field.

Medicine

Key to understanding the current status of nursing research is the profound influence of medical discourse. Medicine has been exceptionally effective at developing a body of abstract knowledge through which it has been able to advance wide-ranging jurisdictional claims. Sociologists of these so-called medicalization processes have drawn attention to their power to control vast areas of social life and render them legitimate subjects of medical interest (Conrad and Schneider, 1980; Zola, 1972; Illich, 1976). Medicine is an example of a hard applied subject (Becher, 1989) and dominated by the biomedical paradigm in which the emphasis is on the mastery of diseases. Such is its power that students are taught it as an unquestionable fact in the course of their training and such explanations are privileged over others. No justification for its precepts is required and, as a consequence, medical socialization processes reinforce the 'correctness' of this particular worldview.

In the UK since its inception, the National Health Service (NHS) has tended to equate health care with medical care. A cursory glance over the so-called health policies in the UK will confirm the relative invisibility of all other care providers (see for example, Strong and Robinson, 1990) and reveal the assumption that the health services and medical agenda are synonymous.

Within this dominant discourse nurses are constituted as subordinate assistants to the medical agenda (Dingwall and Allen, 2001). Not only does this limit the intellectual aspiration of nurses, it underwrites nursing's inferior status in the hierarchy of health care provision. As we described in the Introduction to Part I, Robinson (2002) felt the full weight of medical power when research findings, which called into question the quality of the services offered, were blocked by powerful players who used her nursing status as a warrant for disregarding them.

Professionalism

A further highly influential discourse has been that associated with nursing's claim to professional status. Within nursing, the discourse of professionalism has been aligned with the traits associated with established professions: skill based on theoretical knowledge; an extensive period of education; the theme of public service and altruism; the existence of a code of ethics; insistence upon professional self-regulation; and testing of members' competence for admission to the professions (Goode, 1960). As Rafferty (1996) has observed, nursing has tended to look to medicine as a model of the mature profession. In particular, it has placed considerable emphasis on 'autonomy' as a master professional trait.

The discourse of professionalism underlines nursing's status as an independent discipline with the power to determine the content and scope of its contribution to society and the knowledge base that underpins this work. Historically the claims made about the nursing function have been crafted and re-crafted by nursing leaders in response to the political and cultural climate of the day. For example, at the end of the nineteenth century Mrs Bedford-Fenwick located the defining features of a profession in the technical and scientific skills of nursing based on the model of the medical profession. In more recent years, however, a contrastive rhetoric has been adopted which, whilst retaining medicine as a key point of reference, links claims to professional status with nursing's unique caring role in contradistinction to the curative functions of medicine. The so-called 'new nursing' professional discourse has seen the reconstruction of the nurse–patient relationship in ways which emphasize the unique qualities of patients and the therapeutic potential of nursing work in assisting patients to find meaning in their experiences. Such a framework of understanding has underpinned the call from sections of the nursing leadership for an all qualified nursing workforce and a practitioner-based division of labour in which professional nurses perform all aspects of an individual's care from body care to specialist technical interventions.

In parallel with efforts to define the nursing function, since the latter half of the nineteenth century the profession has also been engaged in developing and defining a body of knowledge it can call its own. The research field is replete with more-or-less self-conscious attempts to constitute the structure of nursing knowledge and, in so doing, construct an intellectual identity for the discipline in order to underpin the profession's status claims. This process has generated epistemological divisions and debates that are crucial to an understanding of the contemporary shape of nursing research and these are explored in detail in Chapter 4.

Managerialism

Managerialism is also central to understanding the state of nursing research. Within this discourse nursing is constructed as a practice-based profession closely aligned with the needs of the service. Resistance to nurse registration at the end of the nineteenth century was in part owing to the threat that this posed to hospitals' control over nursing work. In the absence of a national system of accreditation, nursing skills were not readily transferable and, as a consequence, hospitals enjoyed a local captive labour market. The registrationist proposals threatened to remove this monopoly so that rather than nurses working on terms set by the hospital, the hospitals would have to employ nurses on terms set by the occupation (Dingwall et al., 1988).

In the 1960s, managerialist discourse was actually deployed as a vehicle of occupational advancement by the nursing leadership. When Taylorist philosophies and scientific management[1] were at the height of their popularity in the health care sphere, claims for managerial roles and equality of status with administrators was the strategy by which the health professions other than medicine sought to enhance their status and rewards (Harrison and Pollitt, 1994). In the 1970s the Salmon reforms introduced a structure that was intended to modernize nursing management and achieve a more efficient use of nursing labour. A management structure was implemented which gave nursing parity with other interests in the NHS (Dingwall et al., 1988). However, as Carpenter (1977) points out, although the nursing elite maintained they were attempting to uplift the profession as whole, in reality the gains of Salmon were very narrow. Equality of nursing with other groups in management was won by virtue of the elite's domination over the nursing labour force and did little to ameliorate medical dominance in clinical arena, and this led to considerable disillusionment at the lower levels of the nursing hierarchy.

In the twenty-first century, as part of wider efforts to increase the efficiency of modern health care systems, managerial discourses have focused on nursing skill mix. Rather than the nursing function being defined by the profession, within this discourse its jurisdiction is tied to the changing needs of the service. As the largest occupational group and the single largest item of expenditure in the service, nursing work has been in the spotlight in the search for more cost-effective ways of providing care. They are also the group to whom managers have looked to take on doctor-devolved work in the context of efforts to reduce the hours worked by junior doctors. Whereas professional discourse emphasizes the uniqueness of the client–professional relationship and practitioner autonomy, managerial discourse stresses effectiveness, efficiency, organizational standards, accountability and control.

Gender

Throughout nursing's history, medical, professional and managerial discourses have been infused with the politics of gender, displaying clearly how discourses can be mutually reinforcing. Gendered discourse provides the basis for unequal relationships between men and women on the grounds of their biological differences. Gender has been both a liability and a resource for nurses (Gamarnikow, 1978, 1991; Walby, 1986; Walby and Greenwell, 1994). Garmarnikow (1978, 1991) has argued that the reforms of nursing in the nineteenth century were informed by gendered discourse to which both nurses and doctors subscribed. It was deployed by reformers in order to support the establishment of an occupational niche for single or widowed middle-class women: women ought to do nursing work it was claimed because the tasks involved were identical to those women performed in the domestic sphere and because caring qualities were uniquely feminine. Yet whereas reformers used gendered ideologies in an enabling way, doctors defined femininity in terms of patriarchy. Feminist scholars have drawn attention to the dangers of such explicitly gendered occupational strategies. Women carry into the workplace their status as subordinate individuals and this status comes to define the value of the work that they do (Phillips and Taylor, 1980). If nurses' skills are based on the natural attributes of womanhood why do they necessitate investment in a programme of education and training (Needleman and Nelson, 1988)? It is precisely such gendered thinking which has made progression of the discipline challenging because 'once a field becomes identified in terms of certain characteristics [...] a whole set of properties inherent in that identification come into play – properties which can profoundly affect the way of life of those engaged in the exploration of the field' (Becher, 1989). Here we can see how gendered and managerial discourses can reinforce each other to produce the anti-intellectualism which has been such a prominent feature of nursing's occupational development. There are clear benefits in down-grading the skills required of nurses, given that nurses constitute one of the single largest items of health expenditure. But it is precisely such gendered anti-intellectualism which has, according to some, left nursing today as 'a field of practice without a scientific heritage ... a profession without the theoretical base it seems to require' (Johnson, 1974).

In the following sections and subsequent chapters we examine the impact of these discourses on the shape of nursing research in key arena: education, research policy and practice.

Nurse education policy

Historically, in the UK, the intersection of managerial, medical and gendered discourses has exerted a powerful influence over nurse education despite efforts by leaders of the occupation to advance professional agenda. It is only relatively recently that nursing has entered wholesale into the higher education sector and this happened at a historical moment when professional and managerial agenda converged, albeit briefly. For the most part, nurse education policy has been driven by the need to maintain high student throughput in order to meet service needs and, as a predominantly female occupation, it has been founded on gendered assumptions about the career paths and social roles of women.

Examining nurses' 'professional predicament', Davies (1995) contrasts the high recruitment/high wastage model of womanpower underpinning nurse education with conventional low recruitment/low wastage manpower models. She reveals how in the past student nurses provided a cheap source of labour and skilled assistance to a medical agenda, but it was assumed that many would leave the service (primarily for marriage and child-bearing) and would be replaced by the next cohort. The logical extension of such a model is that there is no need to invest in an expensive initial training, or develop a career structure and opportunities for post-registration continuing professional development.

Although academic departments of nursing have existed since the 1970s, these were the exception rather than the rule. Until the early 1990s, most (98 per cent) nurse education/ training took place in hospital-based schools of nursing, managed by directors of nurse education who were accountable to the health authority. Training was primarily practice-based and summative assessment was by means of national examination which had no academic currency. Short blocks of classroom learning were sandwiched between longer periods of clinical practice. Nursing students were included in hospitals' staff numbers and essential to service delivery. The relationship between nurse education and health service provision was fraught; the needs of the service frequently overshadowing the educational needs of students (Meerabeau, 2001b).

It was against this backdrop that the Project 2000 (UKCC, 1987) reforms of nurse education were conceived. Driven by a professional agenda, its proponents saw it as an opportunity to address nursing's low status, poor retention and lack of a clearly defined area of expertise underpinned by a scientific body of knowledge (Beardshaw and Robinson, 1990). Nurse education was relocated to higher education institutions where academic skills were to be valued and rewarded by a diploma in higher education and learners accorded supernumerary status in the clinical setting. Curricula were redesigned to reflect new nursing ideologies and embraced a range of disciplines rather than being dominated by the biomedical paradigm as had hitherto been the case. The aim was to produce nurses who were 'knowledgeable doers' and could practise 'holistically' in a range of health care settings.

The reform reflected a marriage of convenience between nurse leaders' professional aspirations for changes to the education and structure of nursing and the managerial policy priorities of the government. But its fragility was soon evident. For the profession, Project 2000 was predicated on the assumption of an all registered nursing workforce in order to facilitate 'new nursing' models of holistic patient care. For the Government, it represented an opportunity to make efficiency savings and address other management agenda through the creation of a better educated cadre of professional nurses that could undertake doctor-devolved work, supported by an army of less expensive support workers. Here we can see how medical, management and gendered discourses converged to constitute nurses as extensions of the medical division of labour and caring as unskilled work which safely can be delegated to lower grade staff. Government acceptance of Project 2000 included an important proviso that nurses agree to a new national training structure for health care assistants which seriously undermined the profession's effort to achieve an occupational monopoly over caring work. Even more significant, for current purposes, was the impact of *Working for Patients: Education and Training: Working Paper 10* (Department of Health, 1989). For nurse educationalists, Project 2000 had represented an opportunity to cut loose the historical ties of education to service which would allow educationalists greater control over the profession's knowledge and scope of practice. In the event this opportunity was compromised by the extension of the purchaser/provider model, characteristic of the new public management ethos of the time, to the educational contract. Rather than Project 2000 enabling nurse education to control the structure of its knowledge and practice, it became tied to the service through the introduction of market mechanisms.

Project 2000 was rolled out across the UK throughout the 1990s. By the end of the decade, however, there was mounting public and professional concern about the quality of the new model of pre-registration preparation and these criticisms were expressed in gendered terms. In an article in *The Times* in 1996, Nigella Lawson (1996) argued that the reform of nurse education was misguided. She claimed that it prevented 'natural [but not academic] nurses from pursuing a nursing career and that the new nursing curriculum was an inadequate preparation for the practical demands of the job. Whilst acknowledging the broad range of activities that constitutes nursing work, she argued that the ability to perform these did not rest on intellectual ability. She concludes that nursing 'is an honourable, worthy job; pretending it needs academic status to give it respectability is blunderingly offensive – and silly'. Similar themes were taken up in another UK national newspaper by Richard Horton, the then editor of a leading medical journal: *The Lancet*. Horton (1997) suggests that 'by turning their work into a science akin to medicine [nurses] risk displacing plain and simple (and decidedly non-scientific) caring'. According to Horton, '[t]he personal nurse as patient friend, advocate and skilled carer is worth preserving. Nurses do not need the epithets of specialist, practitioner or assistant to dignify their work. Their status is high enough already. Ask any patient'. In both these articles we can see a common set of themes: that nursing is a moral, rather than a scientific métier; that the work of nurses is 'plain and simple' and that in aspiring to an academic preparation for practice on a par with medicine its members are being silly and getting above their subordinate status as medical assistants. (For a more detailed discussion of these issues see: Allen, 1997; Meerabeau, 2001a.)

These arguments found some favour amidst mounting public concern over standards of basic nursing care. Between 1990 and 1991 the ratio of qualified to unqualified staff shifted from 61:23 to 58:28 (Ranade, 1994). Yet rather than locating the roots of these problems with an increasingly rationalized service, the finger of blame was pointed directly at nurse education. Many argued that nursing was becoming 'too academic' and that insufficient attention was given to practical skills training. It was in this context that the UKCC (United Kingdom Central Council)[2] Commission for Nursing and Midwifery Education was charged with preparing 'a way forward for pre-registration nursing and midwifery education that enables fitness for practice based on health care need'. The Commission reported in 1999 (UKCC, 1999) and whilst acknowledging progress made and the benefits of locating nurse education in institutes of higher education, it also underlined the 'concern that newly qualified nurses, and to a lesser extent midwives, do not possess the practice skills expected of them by their employers'. The solution recommended was 'refocusing pre-registration education on outcomes-based competency principles, to be developed in HEIs in close collaboration with service providers, to ensure that students develop higher order intellectual skills and abilities and the practice knowledge and skills essential to the art and science of nursing and midwifery'.

The response from academic nurses was highly critical. Reflecting on the evidence submitted to the UKCC Education Commission (UKCC, 1999), Mead and Mosley (2000) argue that 'the intellectual skills that help to produce the effective nurses of tomorrow are not valued, or are even denigrated, by politicians and some nurses'. Thompson and Watson (2001) concur, pointing to the ethos pervading nursing in which management discourse and service influences over nurse education have resulted in a system where nurses are encouraged to read, write and think even less and anything perceived to be intellectual is seen as elitist. They suggest that there are people, including those in universities, who would like to see nursing stripped of any pretence at scholarship. It is a moot point as to whether the current system of nurse education is an adequate preparation for practice in modern health services, but such trends clearly contrast sharply with the critical and questioning attitude that characterizes the worldview of researchers which, as Thompson (1998) observes, 'involves creativity, curiosity, and a willingness to take risks'.

Given the dominance of management discourse in shaping nurse education, it is not surprising that it is only relatively recently in the UK that doctoral education has been available for nurses and lags behind the US by some 60 years (McKenna and Galvin, 2004). It was not until nursing moved wholesale into HEIs in the 1990s that nurses began to undertake doctoral study in significant numbers. Furthermore, whereas there has been movement within the international nursing community to identify the bachelor's degree as the basic entry qualification to nursing, and nursing organizations have attempted to raise the status of the profession by campaigning for improvements in preparation for practice, in the UK this has yet to be achieved. For Rafferty and Traynor (1999) it this lack of a graduate education policy for nursing coupled with the deep-seated anti-intellectualism that has plagued the profession that is perhaps the most significant constraint on building research capacity.

Building research capacity within academe

Given this history, it is not surprising that research capacity in academic departments of nursing is so under-developed. Prior to nursing's entry to higher education, nurse teachers, who were based in colleges of nursing, were selected on the basis of their clinical teaching skills rather than their research capability and interest. Thus when nursing made its entry into the higher education sector, few nurse educators were educated to degree and even fewer to masters and doctoral level. Furthermore, the continuing influence of management discourse on nurse education policy has made building research capacity in the sector particularly challenging.

Unlike other disciplines which are funded by the Higher Education Funding Councils, pre-registration nurse education is resourced through health service budgets. No provision is made within educational contracts to develop scholarship and research as part of the nurse lecturer role. Instead the emphasis is on the teaching and practical preparation of large numbers of students in order to meet service needs. In addition to its high volume of students, nurse education is characterized by intensive student contact teaching methods. The teaching year in nurse education spans 45 weeks compared to courses funded by the four Higher Education Funding Councils in which the teaching year is typically 36 weeks. So whereas the summer is an opportunity for academics in other disciplines to concentrate on their research activity, this is not an option for nurses. There is also anecdotal evidence to suggest that nurse lecturers devote more time to the pastoral care of students than is typical of other disciplines. At one level this arises from the need to respond to a range of tensions in nurse education: the wide entry gate to the profession and a high proportion of mature students, the demands of clinical placements and nurse lecturers' gate-keeping role in ensuring clinical safety and fitness for practice. At another level, it might also be seen as the result of the operation of gendered expectations arising from nurses' role in the clinical context, where nurse academics expect, and are expected, to care for others. It is interesting to note that in other disciplines, female academics tend to undertake a greater proportion of pastoral work than male colleagues, and this has been one of a number of identified factors explaining the relative under-performance of women academics (Morley, 1994).

The challenge of building an academic base has been shaped further by state interference in nurse education which, as we have seen, has undergone two major reforms over the last 15 years, requiring rewriting of curricula. Moreover, as the generalist health care professional, nursing work is particularly susceptible to changes in health technologies and wider health policies. It was to nurses that health services managers looked when the European Working

Time Directive made it necessary to review junior doctors' work. It is nursing that will be changed by increasing hospital acuity and the (re)domestication of care and it is through the creation of new nursing roles that policy makers aspire to tackle some of the most intractable problems of the service. Nevertheless, such innovation in workforce planning has not extended to educational policy making, where the current emphasis on competencies is likely to ensure that nursing curricula are even less responsive to the evolving needs of the service. Meerabeau (2001a) attributes this state of affairs to the profession's failure to establish a rigorous intellectual foundation (like social work and unlike medicine) and it is certainly true that nursing struggles to articulate its core functions. Academic nursing is clearly caught in a vicious circle.

Despite the demands of teaching and student support, nurse lecturers face considerable pressure to augment their academic credibility by undertaking doctoral study. The increase in nurses registered for doctoral degrees identified in the mapping of nursing research undertaken by Traynor and Rafferty (1998), can be largely attributed to nurse academics. Despite evidence of progress, at the time of writing it remains far from clear whether the service-driven nature of nurse education will ever permit the development of academic profiles typical of orthodox disciplines. Whilst it ought to be possible to ensure that all university departments of nursing are research informed, it may be that because of the requirement to manage the clinical and academic demands of nursing practice, the sector can only actually support a proportion of staff actively engaged in the production of original research. We consider this issue in greater detail in Chapter 5.

Research capacity in clinical practice

If there are barriers to building research capacity in academe, then the challenges faced by nurses in the clinical domain are even more overwhelming. It is in this context that the power of medical and management discourse is felt most acutely. As a number of commentators have observed (Flynn, 2002; Timmermans and Berg, 2003), evidence-based practice (EBP) is a hybrid form of organizational governance which endeavours to enrol health care professionals into a management agenda (of containing health care costs and standardizing practice) whilst giving them some semblance of delegated autonomy. It represents an attempt to meld management and professional discourses in a single system and as a consequence contains within it some contradictory elements. For some, EBP represents an opportunity for nursing to harness professional aspirations to wider policy trends. For others, EBP confirms the dominance of management discourse which seeks to reduce nursing practice to the unthinking application of best practice guidelines (Freshwater and Rolf, 2004).

There is some evidence for this more pessimistic interpretation. The nursing career structure to support research and development in clinical practice is limited (WAG, 2004) and there is an absence of clear educational pathways to support the development of research leaders. Indeed, it is a powerful indicator of the continued power of medical discourse that it is the research nurse that is the most common clinical research role. Such posts tend to mirror the traditional medical–nursing relationship in which the nurse's contribution is to assist and manage medically driven projects rather than undertake nurse-led work. Reporting findings on a survey undertaken at the University of Manchester, Luker (1999) has drawn attention to the variability in the educational preparation of research nurses in which only 16 out of 77 had had formal training in research methods. This is the research equivalent of the gendered 'adjunct work' (Davies, 1995) performed by their colleagues in the clinical setting.

That is, ill-defined support work that has clear parallels with the work of a wife, and which draws on gendered assumptions about the 'natural' talents of women.

The development of nurse consultant posts in the UK in which research is one of five specified functions is a step in the right direction. However, research is one element in a very full and demanding role which also includes education, management, and clinical work, and tends to be the function that is less well developed and for which incumbents are least well prepared. Job descriptions fail to describe with any degree of specificity the modes of research engagement relevant for the post (see also Chapter 5) and despite being fashioned on the medical consultant model, the role lacks an underpinning infrastructure. Unlike their medical counterparts, nurse consultants do not have a team of juniors to support their work, instead the onus is placed on the leadership skills and personal qualities of individual role incumbents.

Research policy

Rafferty *et al.* (RCN, 2004) trace the fortunes of nursing in UK research policy and in so doing highlight how the dominance of medical discourse has contrived to render invisible the specific needs of nursing *vis-à-vis* the development of its research base. They identify the overlap in the recommendations made in two 'landmark' papers, published seven years apart (Department of Health, 1993b, 2000a) and draw attention to the lack of progress made in the intervening period. They observe that despite the existence of a taskforce document focused on nursing and midwifery research (Department of Health, 1993a) *The Research Capacity Strategy for the Department of Health and the NHS: A First Statement* (Department of Health, 1996) hardly mentions nursing at all. These authors point to the relatively high proportion of the discussion centred on the medical profession as evidence of the fact that the NHS research and development (R&D) was seen primarily as research that is undertaken by doctors. Although an annex is devoted to a consideration of the difficulties facing non-medical professions, no recommendations are made as to how their particular needs might be addressed and no aspects of the strategy specifically consider the requirements of nursing, midwifery and health visiting. Rafferty *et al.* draw the same conclusions from an analysis of the policy documents linked to the clinical governance agenda (Department of Health, 1998, 2000a) and government documents addressing research workforce needs (Department of Health, 1998, 2000a). The Mant Report (Department of Health, 1997) is identified by these authors as an unusual example of a government document that makes recommendations about the specific needs of nurses, midwives and health visitors, but it fails to acknowledge the extent of need, the potential contribution and the actions necessary.

In key documents focused on *nursing*, managerial discourse ensures that the emphasis remains on the needs of the service, and it is *R&D* that receives scant attention. Rafferty *et al.* (2004) analyse the place of R&D in *Making a Difference* (Department of Health, 1999) which sets out the nursing contribution to modernizing the NHS and improving the nation's health. They consider the potential contribution of R&D for each of the key elements in this document and compare this with the actual attention that is received. For example, in the section considering research and training it is the clinical expertise of nurse educators that is given emphasis, underlining the value accorded to practical training over intellectual and academic skills. It is also the case that in the sections on career pathways, leadership and working in new ways, R&D is hardly mentioned. The strongest statement on R&D is in the chapter devoted to clinical quality and the need for critical appraisal skills, research capacity and research career pathways. However, Rafferty *et al.* (2004) conclude: 'nurse researchers might be forgiven for thinking that this single paragraph of intended activity is too insignificant within the document as a whole to permit confidence that a commitment to R&D is integral to *Making a Difference*'.

The power of dominant discourses to render nursing research invisible, is reflected in the fact that in the UK, no single public or funding agency has assumed a responsibility for funding, promoting and coordinating nursing research (Mead and Mosley, 2000). Instead nursing research, like that of the allied health professions, is simply an adjunct to predominantly medical concerns. One of the consequences of the low profile of nursing R&D and the exclusion of nurses from policy-making arena, is that research questions relevant to these professions and/or capacity building have not been integrated into the commissioning strategies of major research funding bodies (Rafferty *et al.*, 2000).

The need to exert an influence over the NHS R&D agenda is a recurrent theme in recent policy documents on nursing research. For example, *Towards a Strategy for Nursing Research and Development: Proposals for Action*, states:

> There are two principal dimensions to influencing the research and development agenda: ensuring the important areas of research about nursing receive appropriate priority: and ensuring that general priority setting benefits from a nursing perspective. The key to the former rests in establishing and asserting credible priorities in appropriate arena. The key to the latter rests in ensuring that there is a well-informed nursing contribution to priority setting exercises and appropriate representation on programme boards, panels and other influential research groups.
>
> (Department of Health, 2000b, p. 3)

Pearson (2000) draws attention to the learnt helplessness and reluctance to engage with the policy processes that can arise from the power of dominant discourses to silence the nursing voice. She warns against 'being so overwhelmed by the sense of enduring systematic exclusion from the mainstream R&D world, that we fail to take responsibility for seizing those opportunities which already exist to make a difference' (Pearson, 2000). A number of nursing organizations have recognized the need to provide training for nurses in the skills required to influence political leaders (WAG, 2004). Recognition of the difficulties experienced by many groups outside medicine in influencing priority-setting exercises has also led the Health Technology Assessment (HTA), a national R&D programme, to launch a consultative exercise led by Professor Foxcroft, aimed at identifying ways of improving the participative processes for agreeing the UK research agenda (Centre for Policy in Nursing Research *et al.*, 2001).

Recent gains in securing targeted investment in nursing R&D in the UK have come as the result of sustained lobbying on the part of representatives of the profession and the convergence of professional and policy agenda. The Department of Health and Higher Education Funding Council (England) doctoral and post-doctoral award schemes, referred to in Chapter 1, were based on the recommendations arising from a task group, chaired by Professor Janet Finch, vice-chancellor of Keele University. The task group's report (HEFCE, 2001) presented a strong case for future investment in nursing research. Rafferty *et al.* (2004) suggest that the task group's case was bolstered by the adoption of an inclusive approach which embraced nursing and allied health professions, and enabled policy makers to tackle several issues with a single solution.

Conclusions

In this chapter we have drawn on the work of Foucault to trace the combined effects of key discourses in different arenas in shaping the contours of nursing research in the UK. As an externally generated discipline, we have seen how academic nursing has been influenced directly and indirectly by wider economic and political interests which have consistently privileged the immediate (practical) needs of the service over longer-term developmental needs. One important consequence of these social processes has been to impoverish the progression of the knowledge base for nursing practice and seriously curtail the profession's capacity for addressing this state of affairs. Furthermore, it has set in train segmentation processes, creating divisions within the knowledge community. The most obvious of these is that which exists between the worlds of practice and academia which has made forging the links between knowledge generation, and utilization a significant challenge.

Notes

1   Scientific management is a set of principles governing the design of jobs which entail the separation of mental from manual labour, sub-division of tasks, de-skilling, close managerial control of work effort and incentive wage payments. The movement originated in the USA, F. W Taylor being its main proponent.
2   The UKCC was replaced in 2002 by the Nursing and Midwifery Council (NMC) under the Nursing and Midwifery Order 2001 (SI 2002/253 (the Order).

References

Allen, D. (1997) 'Nursing, knowledge and practice', *Journal of Health Service Research Policy*, 2, 190–3.
—— (2001) *The Changing Shape of Nursing Practice: The Role of Nurses in the Hospital Division of Labour*, London: Routledge.
Beardshaw, V. and Robinson, R. (1990) *New for Old? Prospects for Nursing in the 1990s*, London: Kings Fund Institute.
Becher, T. (1989) *Academic Tribes and Territories: Intellectual Enquiry and the Cultures of Disciplines*, Milton Keynes: Open University Press.
Carpenter, M. (1977) 'The new managerialism and professionalism in nursing', in M. Stacey, M. Reid, C. Heath and L.R. Dingwall (eds) *Health and the Division of Labour*, London: Croom Helm.
Centre for Policy in Nursing Research, R&D Forum Allied Health Professions, Association of Commonwealth Universities and CHEMS Consulting (2001) *Promoting Research in Nursing, Midwifery, Health Visiting and Allied Health Professions*: Report of the Task Group 3 to HEFCE and the Department of Health. Bristol: Higher Education Funding Council for England.
Conrad, P. and Schneider, J.W. (1980) *Deviance and Medicalization: From Badness to Sickness*, St Louis, MO: C.V. Mosby.
Davies, C. (1995) *Gender and the Professional Predicament in Nursing*, Buckingham: Open University Press.
Department of Health (1989) *Working for Patients. Education and Training. Working Paper 10*, London: Department of Health.
—— (1993a) *Report of the Taskforce on the Strategy for Research in Nursing, Midwifery and Health Visiting*, London: Department of Health.
—— (1993b) *Research for Health*, London: Department of Health.
—— (1996) *Research Capacity Strategy for the Department of Health and the NHS: A First Statement*, London: Department of Health.

—— (1997) *R&D in Primary Care: National Working Group Report* (The Mant Report), London: Department of Health.

—— (1998) *A First Class Service: Quality in the New NHS*, London, Department of Health.

—— (1999) *Making a Difference: Strengthening the Nursing, Midwifery and Health Visiting Contribution to Health and Healthcare*, London: Department of Health.

—— (2000a) *Research and Development for a First Class Service*, Leeds: Department of Health.

—— (2000b) *Towards a Strategy for Nursing Research and Development: Proposals for Action*, London: Department of Health.

Dingwall, R. and Allen, D. (2001) 'The implications of healthcare reforms for the profession of nursing', *Nursing Inquiry*, 8, 64–74.

Dingwall, R., Rafferty, A.M. and Webster, C. (1988) *An Introduction to the Social History of Nursing*, London and New York: Routledge.

Flynn, R. (2002) 'Clinical governance and governmentality', *Health, Risk & Society*, 4, 155–72.

Freshwater, D. and Rolf, G. (2004) *Deconstructing Evidence-Based Practice*, Abingdon: Routledge.

Gamarnikow, E. (1978) 'Sexual division of labour: the case of nursing', in A. Kuhn and A.M. Wolpe (eds) *Feminism and Materialism: Women and Modes of Production*, London: Routledge and Kegan Paul.

—— (1991) 'Nurse or woman: gender and professionalism in reformed nursing 1860–1923', in P. Holden and J. Littleworth (eds) *Anthropology and Nursing*, London: Routledge.

Goode, W. (1960) 'Encroachment, charlatanism, and the emergent professions', *American Sociological Review*, 25, 902–14.

Harrison, S. and Pollitt, C. (1994) *Controlling Health Professionals*, Milton Keynes: Open University Press.

HEFCE (2001) *Research in Nursing and Allied Health Professions: Report of the Task Group 3 to HEFCE and the Department of Health*, London: HEFCE.

Horton, R. (1997) 'Health: a complicated game of doctors and nurses', *The Observer*, 30 March.

Illich, I. (1976) *Limits to Medicine*, London: Marion Boyars.

International Council of Nurses (1997) *Nursing Research: Building International Research Agenda*. Report of the Expert Committee on Nursing Research, Geneva: ICN.

Johnson, D. (1974) 'Development of a theory: a prerequisite for nursing as a primary health profession', *Nursing Research* 23, 372–7.

Lawson, N. (1996) 'Is it the end nurses?', *The Times*, 26 December.

Luker, K.A. (1999) 'The dilemma concerning the nurse's role in a multidisciplinary research agenda', *Nursing Times Research*, 4, 85–6.

McKenna, H. and Galvin, K. (2004) 'Doctoral processes: the scholarly practitioner', in D. Freshwater, and V. Bishop (eds) *Nursing Research in Context: Appreciation, Applications and Professional Developments*. Basingstoke: Palgrave Macmillan.

Mead, D. and Mosley, L. (2000) 'Developing nursing research in a contract-driven arena: inequities and iniquities', *Nursing Standard*, 15, 39–43.

Meerabeau, E. (2001a) 'Back to the bedpans: the debates over preregistration nursing education in England', *Journal of Advanced Nursing*, 34, 427–35.

—— (2001b) 'Can a purchaser be a partner? Nursing education in the English universities', *International Journal of Health Planning and Management*, 16, 89–105.

Morley, L. (1994) 'Glass ceiling or iron cage: women in UK academia', *Gender, Work and Organization*, 1, 194–203.

Needleman, R. and Nelson, A. (1988) 'Policy implications: the worth of women's work', in A. Stratham, E. Miller, H. Mauksch (eds) *The Worth of Women's Work: A Qualitative Synthesis*, New York: State University New York.

Pearson, M. (2000) 'Making a difference through research: how nurses can turn the vision into reality' (Guest Editorial), *Nursing Times Research*, 5, 85–6.

Phillips, A. and Taylor, B. (1980) 'Sex and skill: notes towards a feminist economics', *Feminist Review*, 6, 79–88.

Prior, L. (1989) *The Social Organization of Death: Medical Discourses and Social Practices in Belfast*, London: Macmillan.

Rafferty, A.M. (1996) *The Politics of Nursing Knowledge*, London and New York: Routledge.

Rafferty, A.M. and Traynor, M. (1999) 'Building and benchmarking research capacity for nursing', *Nursing Times Research*, 4, 5–7.

Rafferty, A.M., Bond, S. and Traynor, M. (2000) 'Does nursing, midwifery and health visiting need a research council?', *Nursing Times Research*, 5, 325–35.

Rafferty, A.M., Newell, R. and Traynor, M. (2004) 'Research and development: policy and capacity building', in D. Freshwater and V. Bishop (eds) *Nursing Research in Context: Appreciation, Application and Professional Development*, Basingstoke: Palgrave Macmillan.

Ranade, W. (1994) *A Future for the NHS? Health Care in the 1990s*, London and New York: Longman.

RCN (2004) *Research Ethics*, London: RCN.

Robinson, J. (2002) 'Research for whom: the politics of research and dissemination and application', in A.M. Rafferty and M. Traynor (eds) *Exemplary Research for Nursing and Midwifery*, London: Routledge.

Strong, P. and Robinson, J. (1990) *The NHS Under New Management*, Milton Keynes: Open University Press.

Thompson, D. (1998) 'The art and science in clinical nursing', in B. Roe and C. Webb (eds) *Research and Development in Clinical Nursing Practice*, London: Whurr Publishers.

Thompson, D. and Watson, R. (2001) 'Editorial: Academic nursing – what is happening to it and where is it going?', *Journal of Advanced Nursing*, 36, 1–2.

Timmermans, S. and Berg, M. (2003) *The Gold Standard: The Challenge of Evidence-Based Medicine and Standardization in Health Care*, Philadelphia, PA: Temple University Press.

Traynor, M. (1999) *Managerialism and Nursing*, London and New York: Routledge.

Traynor, M. and Rafferty, A.M. (1998) *Nursing Research and the Higher Education Context: A Second Working Paper*, London: Centre for Policy in Nursing Research, London School of Hygiene and Tropical Medicine.

UKCC (1987) *Project 2000: The Final Proposals*, London: UKCC.

——— (1999) *Fitness for Practice: the UKCC Commission for Nursing and Midwifery* (chair Sir Leonard Peach), London: UKCC.

WAG (2004) *Realising the Potential: Briefing Paper 6: Achieving the Potential Through Research and Development: A Framework for Realising the Potential Through Research and Development in Wales*, Cardiff: Welsh Assembly Government.

Walby, S. (1986) *Patriarchy at Work: Patriarchal and Capitalist Relations in Employment*, Cambridge: Polity Press.

Walby, S. and Greenwell, J. (1994) *Medicine and Nursing: Professions in a Changing Health Service*, London: Sage.

Zola, I. (1972) 'Medicine as an institution of social control', *Sociological Review*, 20, 487–504.

Chapter 3

Expectations of research

Davina Allen and Patricia Lyne

Introduction

According to Mulhall (1997), research 'has become a hallmark for good practice, a symbol of professionalization, a culture in which both practitioners and researchers collude'. Yet such 'collusion' presents significant challenges. Nursing research is situated at the boundary of the worlds of academia and practice where it straddles different cultures and systems of reward and must confront diverse expectations of what it should accomplish. For example, Le May *et al.* (1998) report on a study of nurses' views of research that revealed the range of expectations that exist.

> For practitioners research was seen as improving and developing care whilst also providing the opportunity for evaluation and standardization of practice. [It] gave professional credibility, confidence and justification for staffing levels. [...] For managers research was more instrumental in creating a good image, marking the trust as innovative, and attracting and maintaining dynamic staff – hallmarks of a good organization.
>
> (Le May *et al.*, 1998, p. 431)

This extract contains a range of potentially contradictory expectations of research. It is a tool for service evaluation, a mechanism to support the standardization of practice, a token of professional credibility and source of confidence, a justification for staffing levels, and a marker of a dynamic organization. Beyond such internal requirements others external to the profession – such as policy makers and service managers – have a view of what nursing research should deliver. This state of affairs is by no means unique to nursing, indeed Becher (1989) identifies it as a defining feature of soft applied knowledge fields. He cites the observations of Whitely (1984) that where the central focus of a disciplinary field is largely defined by non-academic groups then its autonomy is constrained and subject to invasion in the name of 'relevance'. This chapter explores the expectations for nursing research, the underlying agenda that drive them and their consequences.

Academic agenda

For certain segments of the occupation, the importance of research lies in its value in underwriting nursing's status claims. The theories and models of nursing that characterized North American nursing research in the late 1970s and 1980s (Tomey and Alligood, 1998) were explicitly linked to a wider professionalization project in which the existence of a theoretical body of knowledge and academic credibility is considered a master professional trait (Goode, 1960). Proponents of this view tend to have their strongest base in university departments of nursing and are more likely to aspire to theoretical, basic and long term research as opposed to applied, evaluative or short-term projects.

A major driver of the work of UK nurse academics is the requirement to secure a high rating in the Research Assessment Exercise (RAE). A department's RAE rating determines the future resources available to it and its standing within the discipline. With each successive RAE, there has been an overall improvement in the ratings received and this has elevated the quality threshold necessary to secure recurrent funding. Academic departments of nursing face particular challenges, because despite nursing's progressive improvement, it lags behind more established disciplines. As funding of research in the UK becomes increasingly selective, in order to secure resources it is necessary to demonstrate, at both individual and departmental level, coherent programmes of research activity of at least international levels of excellence.

Critics have argued that the kinds of research needed to do well in the RAE are rather different from the applied research needed to enhance professional practice and it is claimed that some institutions have had to make a choice between RAE research and NHS research (Centre for Policy in Nursing Research et al., 2001). Expressing concerns that such perceptions might inform behaviour the Higher Education Funding Council for England (HEFCE, 2001) has stressed that the distinction between applied and non-applied research is unhelpful, and notes that the role of research in enabling evidence-based practice and policy making will be difficult to fulfil if support exists only for research of the most direct application (e.g. evaluations of specific treatments). Responding to the concerns of the research community, it is intended that greater effort will be made in the 2008 RAE to establish quality criteria for the assessment of applied research which is to be accorded equal value to other kinds of research. Whilst these arguments are well-taken, it is also the case that tensions do exist between the research agendas of the health service and higher education (HE) and in fact HEFCE admits that funding opportunities may oblige departments to target 'consultancy' research that addresses the immediate needs of the sponsor, rather than aiming to broaden knowledge and understanding. Moreover, the paucity of available research funds for nursing research may encourage academic researchers to respond to the needs of the NHS where funding is available for local projects to address pressing service issues rather than developing a coherent research programme driven by wider scientific questions.

In recognition of these difficulties, in recent years the UK has witnessed an increasing emphasis on HE-NHS partnerships. For example, the Department of Health's document, *Towards a Strategy for Nursing R&D* states that:

> [r]elationships between researchers, educators and practitioners need to be improved as the basis for strategic alliances between individuals and groups from the health service and higher education sectors. It is only through collaborative effort that the research to practice gap can be closed.
>
> (Department of Health, 2000, p. 6)

These are laudable aims, but we have witnessed how these tensions have played out in the context of nurse education (see Chapter 2) and just how easy it will be to realize this future vision for nursing research remains to be seen. For some, 'there is a fundamental disjuncture between the world of research and the world of practice' (Mulhall, 1997).

Practitioner agenda

With the advent of evidence-based practice (EBP) and clinical governance in the UK, research is increasingly becoming a priority for practitioners. In recent years there has been growing concern about the lack of scientific evidence for much of clinical activity. In the most comprehensive study of research to support nurse decision making to date, Thompson *et al.* (2001a, 2001b) conclude that nurses routinely encounter clinical questions for which they do not have answers. This was confirmed by a research scoping exercise undertaken in one of our partner NHS Trusts designed to inform the nursing research and development strategy, which revealed that clinicians' overwhelming concern was how to access evidence to support practice (Satherley and Price, 2002).

It is also the case, however, that many practitioners remain wary of research and the culture which produces it (Mulhall, 1997). Although constrained by the politico-economic requirements of funding bodies, academic researchers do retain a certain freedom to pose particular critical and enquiring research questions which may generate multifaceted and contradictory explanations. In contrast, the service setting is dominated by the medical and management discourses in which the expectation is that research will produce prescriptive theories and provide optimal, unambiguous and consensual answers to practice problems (Chandler, 1991). From the practice perspective, the value of research is as a means to an end: that which does not provide answers for clinical questions is of little relevance to the real world of the NHS. Whereas from an academic perspective, the value of many research projects arises from how they stimulate more reflective and questioning attitudes by extending the way nurses think about what they do and how they relate to the people they care for (Closs and Cheater, 1994).

Whilst the emergence of the reflective practitioner and frameworks for clinical supervision offer some point at which these two worlds might meet, there are clearly important differences of emphasis. There is evidence of anti-academic feeling within the NHS (Traynor and Rafferty, 1998) and the sense that the concerns of academe have little relevance for the work of those at the front-line of service delivery. Le May *et al.* (1998) capture these sentiments in citing a nurse manager who claims that: 'if you were to ask me to give you a picture of a researcher, then a nursing researcher is someone definitely not wearing a uniform, probably walking around with a great pile of books and papers, and somehow the patient is a bit off there' (Le May *et al.*, 1998, p. 432).

There is clearly some substance to this nurse manager's world view. As we describe in Chapter 4, nursing research in the UK has tended to be dominated by academic endogenous nursing concerns rather than the needs of practice and those journals regarded by academics as having high impact and esteem are seen as inaccessible (Traynor *et al.*, 2001) and fail to convince practitioners of their value (Hunt, 1981). It is also the case that much of nursing research has been driven by descriptive rather than explanatory or prescriptive theories, although it might be argued that the former is a necessary precursor to the development of the latter. At a more fundamental level, however, these difficulties arise from the perpetuation of the false expectation that research can provide a definitive answer to practice problems (Tierney, 1987). Whereas the reality is that, at any given time, the research evidence is partial and liable to produce a different interpretation as more data are generated.

> Knowledge has many metaphors. The image of a landscape is only one, another favoured candidate is a seamless cloak. That, however, has implications of continuity and

coherence which bear poor comparison with the current state of human understanding. From the perspective of those engaged in its creation, knowledge would appear more closely comparable with a badly made patchwork quilt some of whose constituent scraps of material are only loosely tacked together, while others untidily overlap, and yet others seem inadvertently to have been omitted, leaving large and shapeless gaps in the fabric of the whole.

(Becher, 1989, p. 7)

Such a difference of understanding is central to the difficulties in bridging the worlds of academia and practice we are discussing and is, in part, responsible for the inability of practitioners to find answers to their practice problems which leads to a distrust of research. It is also the case that recent strategies designed to promote evidence-based nursing practice may have inadvertently heightened these difficulties creating unrealistic expectations of research and practice alike.

To date the EBP agenda within nursing has largely been driven by educators who have tended to emphasize the 'professional' rather than the 'managerial' rationalities in the EBP hybrid (see Chapter 2). 'Professional' versions of EBP take their lead from Sackett *et al.* (1996) in which it is defined as the 'conscientious and judicious use of current best evidence in making decisions about the care of individual patients'. Accordingly, much of the focus of activity has concentrated on equipping nurses with the skills necessary to utilize research and this has typically entailed critical appraisal skills training and an introduction to the process of conducting research. The 'professional' model of EBP stresses the agency of individual practitioners. French (1999) provides a good example, in the nursing context. Here EBP is defined as: 'The systematic interconnecting of scientifically generated evidence with the tacit knowledge of the expert practitioner to achieve change in a particular practice for the benefit of a well defined client/patient group'. This is a vision in which EBP becomes a tool of local professional autonomy: front line staff accessing the available research in order to make practice decisions or develop services based on the best available evidence. It is becoming increasingly clear, however, that such a model contains within it considerable challenges and that alternative approaches may be called for.

Evaluating and synthesizing a body of evidence is a lengthy process requiring specialist skills to undertake the process rigorously. Closs and Cheater (1994) have suggested that converting research into practical nursing actions needs to be a collaborative responsibility and engage research specialists, clinicians and managers. A further difficulty is that the model is predicated on misguided assumptions about the utilization of evidence in practice. Founded as it is on professional discourses which stress the autonomy of individual practitioners, it ignores the daily reality of much nursing practice, in which nurses work in teams (Allen, 2002). Thompson *et al.* (2001a) found that it was the human sources of research-based information that were overwhelmingly seen by nurses of all levels of educational attainment as the most accessible (physically and intellectually) (see also Tjora, 2000).

As a result of increasing understanding of the complexities of getting evidence into practice, alternatives to the professional model of EBP are emerging. Thompson *et al.* (2001b) suggest that the highest organizational returns for those seeking to make research-based information accessible are likely to be derived from strategies which harness the power of human change agents – such as clinical nurse specialists and consultant nurses. The authors stop short of describing the characteristics of such a research function but underline the importance of adequate educational preparation. This is a rather different model of EBP in which evidence-based knowledge is located in specific roles, rather than being the preserve of all nurses.

Closs and Cheater (1994) point to the lessons learnt from the CURN (Conduct and Utilization of Research in Nursing) project (USA) which recognized the need for research utilization to be framed as an organizational process, rather than the responsibility of individual practitioners. The activities making up this process included the identification and synthesis of research findings; the translation of research-based knowledge into a solution or clinical protocol; the transformation of the clinical protocol into specific nursing actions, and an evaluation of the practice. The organizational approach to research utilization was put into operation by means of a committee which acted as a group of change agents which had both formal and informal links with the practice areas. Closs and Cheater conclude that the assumption that research implementation is the province of the researcher or the individual practitioner, at clinical or managerial level, rather than being part of an organizational process, involving people at all levels is increasingly being discounted (Bircumshaw, 1990; Funk *et al.*, 1991; Horsley *et al.*, 1983; Hunt *et al.*, 2001; McGuire, 1990).

Management agenda

From the perspective of service managers research has several functions. The most obvious is its role in ensuring consistency in the delivery of high quality, cost-effective health care services. In the UK NHS an unprecedented emphasis has been placed on evidence: professional expertise is no longer a guarantor of quality and government policies make it very clear that its aim is to rid the service of inexplicable variations in practice. The launch of the clinical governance framework pointed to a future in which evidence-based national standards and guidelines would be developed to inform practice and organizations would be held to account for any variation in meeting these benchmarks. *A First Class Service* (Department of Health, 1998) identifies two central components being necessary to ensure evidence-based practice is achieved. These are that 'evidence-based practice is supported and applied routinely in everyday practice' and that 'programmes aimed at meeting the needs of individual health care professionals and the service needs of the organization are in place and supported locally'. More recently, integrated care pathways, which – theoretically at least – incorporate evidence-based guidelines, are emerging as the preferred organizational technology to support service improvement.

Despite insistence that individual professional expertise is central to the evidence-based practice agenda many practitioners view the development of guidelines as 'cookbooks' which promote an unthinking adherence to protocols. Many believe they 'are an attempt to erode practitioner autonomy, an aspiration which may also be construed as consonant with liberal ideology which opposes the power of professional elites' (Colyer and Kamath, 1999). EBP has also been criticized for failing to recognize the realities and complexities of clinical practice (Greenhalgh, 1996), many aspects of which do not lend themselves to the formulation of single answerable questions or the application of discrete, definitive interventions. One major source of debate has centred on the dominant approach to systematic reviews of the literature which hitherto has been based on a strictly enforced hierarchy of evidence, with the randomized control trial (RCT) as the so-called 'gold standard'. The elevation of experimental research to a superior position in terms of the quality and applicability to health care practice has been questioned by researchers and practitioners alike. Whilst the RCT provides the best evidence of effectiveness, health professionals are concerned with more than cause and effect questions (Pearson, 2004). More recently a more comprehensive approach to secondary evidence has started to develop, with several groups working on the development of rigorous methods for the review and synthesis of a wider range of methods (Dixon-Woods *et al.*, 2005; Dixon-Woods *et al.*, 2001; Noblit and Hare, 1998; Popay *et al.*, 1998; Popay and Williams, 1998; Lyne *et al.*, 2002).

From a management perspective, research also has value in informing local service development. Increasingly there is an expectation within the NHS that all new services should be evaluated, and this can be an important means of raising the profile of groups and promoting the organization. However, there can sometimes be a mismatch between the kinds of research which are acceptable for organizational purposes and those which meet the quality standards required in academia. For example, evaluation studies of health service interventions present considerable methodological challenges. A number of recent reviews of evaluation studies revealed that these are frequently of poor quality and are neither designed nor reported in ways which lend themselves to transferability (Lyne *et al.*, 2000). In a similar vein, focus group methodology is becoming an increasingly popular method for researching users' experiences, despite the well-documented social scientific critiques which have been directed at their reliability (see for example Dingwall, 1999). From the academic perspective, service managers do not appreciate the requirements of high quality research. From the managers' perspective, however, the research community seems unable to find a cost-effective way of meeting the information needs of the service.

The recent piloting of the 'Safer Patient Initiative' (The Health Foundation 2004) within four UK hospitals is an example of the kind of work that is seen as really helpful within organizations. It depends on the identification, by practitioners, of the many small changes which are needed to improve patient safety, followed by incremental action to bring them about. These changes are made by one nurse, one doctor or one ward at first and then rolled out progressively. No great claims of academic rigour are made for this process, but it appears to be very popular with managers as a means of dealing with patient safety issues. Perhaps more debate is needed between the management and research communities about the nature of 'good enough' evidence.

Policy agenda

Nursing research is also fashioned by the expectations and wishes of policy makers who exercise considerable control over research funding and the setting of research priorities (see Chapter 2). From this perspective, the role of research is to inform the effective development of health services in order to meet future 'need'. Health care problems are not self-evident, however, they have to be conceptualized in a certain way and it is the NHS Central Research and Development Committee that identifies (and effectively defines) research priorities for the NHS and targets areas where information is required (Colyer and Kamath, 1999). The research commissioned clearly reflects wider political concerns and government-defined priorities and, as we saw in the preceding chapter, it has proven very difficult for nursing to influence this agenda, where cost and clinical effectiveness have tended to take precedence over process and quality issues. Moreover, policy makers, for the most part do not have an intimate familiarity with the nature of research, and do not always have an informed appreciation of its relationship with practice or what it can do. This can often result in the production of unwieldy commissioning briefs which, whilst reflecting pressing policy concerns, do not translate well into researchable questions and are often not feasible in practice. In such circumstances securing coveted research funding can be a mixed blessing.

A relatively recent feature of research in the UK is for commissioners to require user involvement in the projects they fund. As part of a wider managerial trend concerned with promoting greater public engagement in social policy in order to counter the power of professional groups within society, it is increasingly an expectation that provision be made for service user involvement in the research process. Whilst in certain instances this is an entirely appropriate aspiration, in others, it may add little to the quality of the endeavour and there is evidence to suggest that the models of citizenship on which such aspirations are based exist more firmly in the minds of politicians than amongst UK citizens. Anecdotally, researchers report project nightmares in which they have found it extremely difficult to institute the ambitious and laudable aspirations for user involvement they have built into their proposals in order to satisfy the requirements of funding bodies. Rather than insisting on user-involvement in the research process, it might be more appropriate to involve them at an earlier stage in the setting of research priorities. Beyond this, the academic principles of the RAE do not lend themselves to research with a strong user involvement. If a researcher were to pursue the strong mode to a possible ultimate position where he or she is facilitating the research user to write the report, or to use the knowledge gained to make a significant change within an organization or take action differently, without a report being written, there would be no brownie points in the RAE. Written outputs of the kind demanded by the RAE are essentially an academic device. The whole process of journal publishing including peer review and great competition for publication means that 'relevant' pieces of work can be dated before they become published (Lewis, 2000).

Many academic researchers have also expressed concern at the increasingly instrumental approach to research in the UK which, it is argued, is progressively undermining the traditional independence of HEIs from government. Drawing on the work of Robert Nisbet (1971), Porter (1997) refers to this process as the 'denigration of academic dogma'. According to Nisbet 'academic dogma' was born amongst the rationalist philosophers of Ancient Greece, which stated that 'all knowledge is good'. What was most valued in academic work was not its immediate usefulness but its contribution to humanity's understanding of itself and of nature. In contrast Nisbet saw the encroachment into mid-twentieth century universities of what he termed academic entrepreneurs, engaged in the sale of knowledge designed for instrumental use. This he saw as a denigration of academic values. Porter suggests that a similar process may be occurring in nursing academia, as part of a broader trend within the higher education sector.

Lewis (2000) raises similar concerns in her commentary on David Blunkett's Economic and Social Research Council (ESRC) lecture in which he called on the academic community to do better and more relevant research. He expresses frustration caused by a tendency for research 'to address issues other than those which are central and directly relevant to the political and policy debate; to fail to take account of the reality of many people's lives; and sometimes to be driven by ideology paraded as intellectual inquiry or critique' (Blunkett, 2000). As Lewis observes, these views suggest a minister firmly in the 'research to provide information' camp, rather than 'research as a contribution to increasing knowledge and understanding' and a straightforward and perhaps rather simplistic view of the relationship between research and policy making. Lewis points out that a real danger of assumptions such as this is that capacity to fund research which has no obvious utility will be lost and the academic community will be increasingly servicing research agenda specified by people who are not researchers and will become reduced to the status of jobbing researchers. She argues that the history of intellectual inquiry is full of examples of intellectual breakthroughs that came about through research which started with no expectation that the researchers would address the issue that emerged.

Conclusion

In this chapter we have traced some of the diverse and contradictory expectations of nursing research and different cultures and structures of rewards which characterize the worlds with which nurse researchers interact. We have noted the different metaphors deployed by users and generators of research to describe the field of knowledge, revealing important differences of perspective. We have shown, too, how the EBP agenda has compounded further this divide. Diverse expectations of the research enterprise are by no means unique to nursing. Gibbons (1985), writes of: 'the tension between the way science (or knowledge) is used in our societies and the way in which it is supposed to be generated'. The challenge for nursing is that these tensions cut across a knowledge community which is itself internally segmented.

References

Allen, D. (2002) 'Time and space on the hospital ward: Shaping the scope of nursing practice', in D. Allen and D. Hughes (eds) *Nursing and the Division of Labour in Healthcare*, Basingstoke: Macmillan Palgrave.

Becher, T. (1989) *Academic Tribes and Territories: Intellectual Enquiry and the Cultures of Disciplines*, Milton Keynes: Open University Press.

Bircumshaw, D. (1990) 'The utilization of research findings in clinical nursing practice', *Journal of Advanced Nursing*, 15, 1272–80.

Blunkett, D. (2000) 'Influence or irrelevance: can social science improve government?', *Secretary of State's ESRC Lecture*, London: ESRC/DofEE.

Centre for Policy in Nursing Research, R&D Forum Allied Health Professions, Association of Commonwealth Universities and CHEMS Consulting (2001) *Promoting Research in Nursing, Midwifery, Health Visiting and Allied Health Professions*: Report of the Task Group 3 to HEFCE and the Department of Health. Bristol: Higher Education Funding Council for England.

Chandler, J. (1991) 'Reforming nurse education: the reorganisation of nursing knowledge', *Nurse Education Today*, 11, 83–8.

Closs, J. and Cheater, F. (1994) 'Utilization of nursing research: culture, interest and support', *Journal of Advanced Nursing*, 19, 762–73.

Colyer, H. and Kamath, P. (1999) 'Evidence-based practice: a philosophical and political analysis: Some matters for consideration by professional practitioners', *Journal of Advanced Nursing*, 29, 188–93.

Department of Health (1998) *A First Class Service: Quality in the New NHS*, London: Department of Health.

—— (2000) *Towards a Strategy for Nursing Research and Development: Proposals for Action*, London: Department of Health.

Dingwall, R. (1999) 'Do focus groups provide all the answers?', *Journal of Health Services Research & Policy*, 4, 191.

Dixon-Woods, M., Fitzpatrick, R. and Roberts, K. (2001) 'Including qualitative research in systematic reviews: Opportunities and problems', *Journal of Evaluation and Clinical Practice*, 7, 125–33.

Dixon-Woods, M., Agarwal, S., Jones, D., Young, B. and Sutton, A. (2005) 'Synthesising qualitative and quantitative evidence: A review of possible methods', *Journal of Health Services & Research Policy*, 10, 45–53.

French, P. (1999) 'The development of evidence-based nursing', *Journal of Advanced Nursing*, 29, 72–8.

Funk, S.G., Champagne, M.T., Wiese, R.A. and Tornquist, E.M. (1991) 'BARRIERS: the barriers to research utilization scale', *Applied Nursing Research*, 4, 39–45.

Gibbons, R. (1985) 'Academic criticism and contemporary literature', in G. Graff and R. Gibbons (eds) *Criticism in the University*, Evanston, IL: Northwestern University Press.

Goode, W. (1960) 'Encroachment, charlatanism, and the emergent professions', *American Sociological Review*, 25, 902–14.

Greenhalgh, T. (1996) 'Is my practice evidence-based?', *British Medical Journal*, 313, 957–8.

HEFCE (2001) *Promoting Research in Nursing and the Allied Health Professions: Research Report 01/64*, London: Higher Education Funding Council England.

Horsley, J.A., Crane, J., Crabtree, M.K. and Wood, D.J. (1983) *Using Research to Improve Nursing Practice: A Guide*, New York: Grune & Stratton.

Hunt, J. (1981) 'Indicators for nursing practice: the use of research findings', *Journal of Advanced Nursing*, 6, 189–94.

Hunt, K., Emslie, C. and Watt, G. (2001) 'Lay constructions of a family history of heart disease: potential for misunderstandings in the clinical encounter?', *The Lancet*, 357, 1168–71.

Le May, A., Mulhall, A. and Alexander, C. (1998) 'Bridging the research-practice gap: Exploring the research cultures of practitioners and managers', *Journal of Advanced Nursing*, 28, 428–37.

Lewis, J. (2000) 'Funding social science research in academia', *Social Policy and Administration*, 34, 365–76.

Lyne, P., Satherley, P. and Allen, D. (2000) *Systematic Review: Effectiveness of Interventions Designed to Reduce or Remove the Barriers to Change to Improve Interagency Working*, Cardiff: University of Wales College of Medicine.

Lyne, P., Allen, D., Satherley, P. and Martinsen, C. (2002) 'Improving the evidence base for practice: a realistic method for appraising evaluations', *Journal of Clinical Effectiveness in Nursing*, 6, 81–8.

McGuire, J.M. (1990) 'Putting research findings into practice: research utilization as an aspect of the management of change', *Journal of Advanced Nursing*, 15, 614–20.

Mulhall, A. (1997) 'Nursing research: our world not theirs?', *Journal of Advanced Nursing*, 25, 969–76.

Nisbet R. (1971) *The Degradation of the Academic Dogma: The University in America 1945–1970*, London: Heinemann.

Noblit, G. and Hare, R. (1998) *Meta-Ethnography: Synthesising Qualitative Studies*, Newbury Park, CA: Sage.

Pearson, A. (2004) 'Balancing the evidence: incorporating the synthesis of qualitative data into systematic reviews', *JBI Reports*, 2, 45–64.

Popay, J. and Williams, G. (1998) 'Qualitative research and evidence-based healthcare', *Journal of Royal Society of Medicine*, 91, 32–7.

Popay, J., Rogers, A. and Williams, G. (1998) 'Rationale and standards for the systematic review of qualitative literature in health services research', *Qualitative Health Research*, 8, 341–51.

Porter, S. (1997) 'Editorial: The degradation of the academic dogma', *Journal of Advanced Nursing*, 25, 655–6.

Sackett, D.L., Rosenberg, W., Gray M.C., Muir, J.A., Haynes, R., Richardson, B. and Scott, W. (1996) 'Evidence based medicine: what is it and what it isn't', *British Medical Journal*, 312, 71–2.

Satherley, P. and Price, M. (2002) *Research and Development: Nursing, Midwifery and Health Visiting Priorities Setting Exercise*, Cardiff: Cardiff and Vale NHS Trust Report.

The Health Foundation (2004) World Health Organization: Launch of the World Alliance for Patient Safety, Washington, DC. Oct 27, 2004, The Health Foundation.

Thompson, C., McCaughan, D., Cullum, N., Sheldon, T., Mulhall, A. and Thompson D. (2001a) 'The accessibility of research-based knowledge for nurses in United Kingdom acute care settings', *Journal of Advanced Nursing*, 36, 11–22.

—— (2001b) 'Research information in nurses' clinical decision-making: what is useful?', *Journal of Advanced Nursing*, 36, 376–88.

Tierney, A.J. (1987) 'Research issues: putting research to good use', *Senior Nurse*, 6, 10.

Tjora, A.H. (2000) 'The technological mediation of the nursing-medical boundary', *Sociology of Health and Illness*, 22, 721–41.

Tomey, A.M. and Alligood, R. (eds) (1998) *Nursing Theorists and their Work*, St Louis, MO: Mosby.

Traynor, M. and Rafferty, A.M. (1998) *Nursing Research and the Higher Education Context: A Second Working Paper*, London: Centre for Policy in Nursing Research, London School of Hygiene and Tropical Medicine.

Traynor, M., Rafferty, A. and Lewinson, G. (2001) 'Endogenous and exogenous research? Findings from a bibliometric study of UK nursing research', *Journal of Advanced Nursing*, 34, 212–22.

Whitely, R. (1984) *The Intellectual and Social Organisation of the Sciences*, Oxford: Clarendon Press.

Chapter 4

The research field

Davina Allen and Patricia Lyne

Introduction

In his analysis of academic tribes and their territories, Becher (1989) observes that: 'the attitudes, activities and cognitive styles of groups of academics representing a particular discipline are closely bound up with the characteristics and structures of the knowledge domains with which such groups are professionally concerned'. So how might we describe the features which characterize the field of nursing research?

Nursing is a segmented and loosely knit cognitive community which crosses, and is shaped by, national cultures. Over the last century the main drivers for research have been its perceived value in contributing to a field of knowledge to underpin the occupation's wider public claims to professional status and its importance in legitimating entry into higher education. One consequence of this is that nursing's disciplinary development has been inextricably bound up with wider professionalization processes. Competing assertions about nursing knowledge have shaped the claims made about its professional identity and different conceptualizations of the nursing function have fashioned epistemological and methodological debates within the discipline. As an applied and externally generated field, nursing research is exposed to more outside interference than is the case for internally generated pure subjects and, as an emergent discipline, it is also faced with the challenge of carving out its intellectual niche in a landscape which is already populated by more established academic tribes. Nursing scholarship is marked by debates about what kind of entities exist, what is considered valid knowledge and how this can be realized. Such ontological and epistemological deliberations have been overlaid by disagreements about whether it should be developing an exclusive body of knowledge or whether it should be looking to apply the insights and methods from other fields.

Central to an understanding of nursing's intellectual development has been its evolving relationship with medicine. As an archetypal profession in a cognate discipline that enjoys high status in the disciplinary pecking order, medicine has been a key point of reference for nursing's self-understanding (see Chapter 2). Historically dependent on doctors for a large part of its education and training, a key thread of nursing's recent professionalizing project has been the establishment of epistemological demarcation and the creation of a knowledge base that is independent from medicine. Segments of the occupation have attempted to establish a separate intellectual and jurisdictional domain through the construction of professional differentiation based on the caring-curing distinction. What has emerged is a holistic biopsychosocial model which places the quality of relationships with clients at the heart of the occupation's public claims to expertise (Aldridge, 1994; Allen, 2001; Salvage, 1992).

A corollary of these developments has been movement away from a traditional dependence on (hard) natural science disciplines to embrace approaches associated with (soft) social scientific disciplines (see for example Holmes, 1990) and in some areas to develop avowedly exclusive nursing epistemologies (Parse, 1981, 2000; Rogers, 1980, 1992; Fawcett, 2000a, 2000b). In this chapter, we review this knowledge field to explore the topics nurse researchers study (and also those they do not), the methods they utilize and their relationships with other disciplines.

What do nurses study?

A considerable proportion of nursing research is endogenous in character. Traynor *et al.* (2001) report on a bibliometric analysis of nursing research outputs in the UK and note that a large proportion of this work is concerned with problems and issues to do with nursing as a profession (including education and pedagogy), as opposed to the 'exogenous' concerns of nursing patients. Solanti (2002) makes similar observations in the context of midwifery research. Traynor *et al.* suggest that this particular feature of the research field may reflect the upsurge in nurse educators undertaking PhDs in subjects relevant to their occupations and the fact that endogenous research is also less resource intensive than exogenous projects. They also propose that endogenous research, focused as it is on the characteristics of nursing, has 'provided a medium for consciousness raising and self-definition for the profession – or at least for groups within it'. The authors argue that it is possible to see parallels in this respect between nursing and other disciplinary groups.

> In the academy, many now relatively established disciplines describe how they have emerged from a period of low levels of articulated debate and little theoretical development. Among them are art and architectural history (Watkin, 1980), literature (Eagleton, 1983, Graeff, 1987), education (Charles, 1988), sociology (Bulmer, 1987), anthropology (De Waal Malefit, 1974), and social policy (Craig, 1997). It seems likely that some of these emerging disciplines have looked to research and a visible intellectual base partly as a means of improving their social and professional status, but also as a way of gaining a systematic understanding of the character and the boundaries of what practitioners in those fields actually do. The articulations of the problems and projects envisaged by some of these groups bear a striking resemblance to those set out within nursing.
>
> (Traynor *et al.*, 2001, p. 220)

It is also the case that, as well as being emergent, the disciplines listed by Traynor *et al.* are examples of soft, and in many cases, also applied disciplines. Becher (1989) argues that in the academic world hard knowledge domains are regarded more highly than soft ones, and pure disciplines are esteemed over applied. He argues that such perceptions are shared to a certain extent by the outside world and that in the competitive environment of knowledge systems, the establishment of a strong academic image is important for external credibility and status. Thus as well as providing a vehicle for developing disciplinary self-understanding, these so-called endogenous activities can also be read as a reflection of a wider need for emergent disciplines to compete in a Darwinian struggle for status and power within the academic system.

Beyond endogenous research, almost all areas of nursing, midwifery and health visiting have generated research activity, very often driven by the imperative of demonstrating the value of nursing and the legitimacy of the professional mandate. Some (e.g. mental health, health promotion) have a longer history than others. In more general terms nurse researchers have demonstrated a particular concern with understanding the experiences of service users and there is a large body of work in this sphere that has emerged in recent years, led by North American and Canadian nurse researchers. Clinically, the emphasis has been in areas where the nursing role is very clear and uncontested, e.g. wound care, promotion of continence, sleep, comfort, pain management, with midwives making early progress in areas such as breast feeding and perineal care (again reflecting a clear understanding of their jurisdiction). Now, as nurses take up specialist responsibilities (such as diabetes, asthma, Parkinson's disease and cancer care) attention is becoming focused on these clinical specialisms and we see the emergence of distinct fields of study within the broad area of nursing research. So the whole field is dynamic and we should not be surprised to see new and distinct disciplines emerging from it, in the same way as other major fields have evolved. For example, irrespective of the debates over science and technology, it is evident that interaction between practical experience, theoretical advances and forces in society have led to the growth and evolution of the constituent disciplines of the natural and physical sciences. From the natural philosophy of the late middle ages, with its combination of religion and mathematics, emerged the parent disciplines of chemistry, physics and biology which in turn have fragmented and combined to produce new disciplines, such as genetics and immunology, with their sub-disciplines, which may eventually branch off from their parents.

There are also some interesting areas which nurses have chosen not to study. Nurses have considerable practice knowledge about bodies and embodiment and yet there has been relatively little nursing research in this area and the field has been left open to colonization by other disciplines (see for example Monaghan, 2001). Julia Lawton's (Lawton, 2000) sociological study of the dying process in a UK hospice sent shock-waves throughout the palliative care community because of the unflinching way in which she describes bodily deterioration. Nurses acquire this knowledge through their practice experience but they have rarely chosen to study it and it remains a largely invisible aspect of the role. A further poorly researched area of nursing practice is the profession's contribution to the people processing and coordinating work of health service organizations. There is ample evidence of the centrality of the importance of this aspect of the nursing function in broader observational studies of health care settings (Allen, 2004; Latimer, 2000), but as yet it has not been identified as a legitimate area of study in its own right.

Certain fields have been inaccessible to nurses because they demand skills which are not common in the profession, for example, those of the laboratory scientist or the epidemiologist. In her commentary on the results of the 2001 RAE, Professor Senga Bond commented on the virtual absence of laboratory based work in the nursing submissions (Bond, 2002). This situation is slowly changing, with nurses developing expertise in areas such as neurophysiology (Carter-Snell and Hegadoren, 2003) tissue engineering (Fader et al., 2004) and wound physiology (Voegeli et al., 1999). As we consider in more detail below, some would argue that such work no longer constitutes 'nursing' but falls under the umbrella of the parent discipline. The counter-argument is that nurses working in such a capacity form a vital bridge between the science and its application by clinicians, and that their involvement with the science stems from their nursing practice in areas such as mental health, continence promotion and wound care.

Approaches to nursing research

Despite these omissions, the contemporary research field is characterized by a breadth of concerns (biopsychosocial), a multiplicity of paradigms, methods and disciplinary approaches. This is entirely fitting, given the scope of the nursing contribution to modern health care systems. Celebrating diversity as one of the strengths of nursing research, Traynor *et al.* (2001) argue that nursing should develop and promote a wide range of methods and approaches to research which bring into view the 'full range of the complex effect of good nursing intervention' (Traynor *et al.*, 2001). Whilst we concur with Traynor *et al.*'s advocacy of intellectual eclecticism, it does bring with it some attendant challenges. The broad church of nursing research is characterized by schisms, sects, charismatic leaders, and acolytes. Many texts display a preoccupation with epistemological demarcation which can lead to overdrawn contrasts between different research approaches. Whilst such sharp distinctions are often fashioned for rhetorical purposes, they are not helpful in promoting an understanding of research methods or the intellectual development of the profession. An obvious example can be found in the field of mental health nursing, where disputes about whether the legitimate basis of nursing practice should be pharmaceutical and psychological interventions or therapeutic relationship building, have become overlaid with debates about the relative value of soft or hard research methods. As a member of the former camp, Gournay (1999) has bemoaned the lack of high quality experimental research in nursing and is critical of its over-reliance on qualitative methods, which he claims are often poorly executed. For Gournay, the future of nursing research would be better served by a shift to quantitative methodologies.

> We [...] argue that there is a history of research largely conducted on nurses and the nature of nursing. Much of this work uses methods that are completely unacceptable to any conventional research discipline. Many published 'research' studies amount to no more than anecdotal accounts of nurses' and patients' experiences. Modern mental health services have complex problems that demand skilfully designed studies, executed with rigour and utilizing batteries of valid and reliable outcome measures.
>
> (Gournay and Ritter, 1997, p. 441)

An example of a position on the other side of the divide can be found in an article by Cutcliffe and Goward (2000) who, in formulating mental health nursing in terms of the centrality of therapeutic relationship building, point to the affinity of mental health nursing to qualitative research and go so far as to suggest that in developing therapeutic relationships with their patients, mental health nurses are engaged in qualitative research.

> [P]sychiatric/mental health nurses are drawn to the qualitative paradigm as a result of the potential synchronicity and linkage that appears to exist between the practice of mental health nursing and qualitative research. The apparent synchronicity appears to centre around the three themes of: (a) the purposeful use of self; (b) the creation of an interpersonal relationship; and (c) the ability to accept and embrace ambiguity and uncertainty. [...] Further it is possible that each nursing situation where the mental health nurse forms a relationship and attempts to gain an empathic sense of the individual's world is akin to an informal phenomenological study, the product of which would be a wealth of qualitative data.
>
> (Cutcliffe and Goward, 2000, p. 590)

Although these seemingly entrenched positions may be over-stated in the literature – with concessions and compromise being acknowledged in the backstage regions of academe – they present real challenges to the novice researcher. Moreover, in our view, whilst philosophical debates about the professions' identity and purpose are to be applauded, these should not be allowed to confound debates about methods appropriate to the investigation of the breadth of nursing concerns. As Johnson (1999) and Johnson *et al.* (2001) have observed, there is a real danger that the models and theories which emerge from such processes become dogma rather than tools to be used critically for thought. What is needed is recognition of the strengths and weakness of all research paradigms and the knowledge which arises from them. Nevertheless, whilst there is no intrinsic scholarly merit in some knowledge forms over others, there does appear to be a preference for studies which entail simple and uncontentious measurement over those which comprise complex and contestable judgements. Given the context in which funding for health care research is available, and the gendered discourses which have shaped nursing's occupational and intellectual development, it is understandable why some segments of the profession would wish to push the case for an orientation of the discipline towards a harder knowledge form as a tactic to strengthen the status and image of the discipline. In Chapter 1 we noted the success of lobbying in the US context in establishing a National Center for Nursing Research within the National Institutes of Health (NIH). Part of the success of the Center can be attributed to the skills of its originators in learning to speak the language of the NIH. This provides a good example of how dominant discourses can be appropriated for professional purposes. Regarded by some as the height of official recognition of the value of nursing research, for others, the turn towards science and a clinical focus on individual patient outcomes came at the expense of much needed research focused on health care systems and wider macro and political issues in health care (Rafferty, 1995).

Primary or secondary discipline?

Each discipline has its linguistic, conceptual and methodological traditions which serve to locate researchers as they formulate their questions and interpretations (Ray, 1999). Such scholarly traditions are central in shaping the ways in which problems are framed. One of the challenges for nursing has been to find its disciplinary voice. Should nursing research be built on conceptual and theoretical foundations which are unique to nursing, or should it be looking to see what can be learnt and applied to nursing from developments in more established fields?

For Mulholland (1997), nursing knowledge is a secondary knowledge form comprising of different primary epistemes. From this perspective, nursing does not possess an independent knowledge base and has a 'situational dependency' on other disciplines. Mulholland draws on Hirst (1975), who makes it clear that nursing is by no means unique in this respect: medicine and engineering are other good examples.

> What there are in abundance now, are new interdisciplinary areas of study in which different forms of knowledge are focused on some particular interest, and because of the relations between the forms, what is understood in each discipline is thereby deepened. Such new areas of study do not constitute new areas on a map of knowledge [...] They are essentially composite, second order forms of knowledge.
>
> (Hirst, 1975, p. 295)

There are, however, people within the field of nursing research that argue strongly that nursing science should be unique to the profession. They reject any dependency on other disciplinary knowledge: any work undertaken within nursing that is informed by disciplines other than nursing is, from this perspective, illegitimate.

> I define nursing research as the generation and testing of empirical nursing theories that are derived from conceptual models of nursing, preferably by means of nursing discipline-specific empirical research methods [...]. I do not regard research done by nurses that generates or tests theories within the context of intellectual traditions from other disciplines as nursing research [...] To think that all research conducted by nurses necessarily is nursing research poses great danger to the advancement of nursing science and the survival of the discipline.
>
> (Fawcett, 2000b, p. 3)

> If mental health is to develop as a distinct discipline, then it requires its own unique knowledge base and its own unique methodologies for adding to that knowledge base.
>
> (Rolfe, 1997, p. 446)

> [N]ursing needs its own unique knowledge base and must take responsibility for developing this, rather than drawing on knowledge from other disciplines, relying on other professional groups and a generic R&D agenda.
>
> (RCN, 2004, p. 3)

The need for caution in drawing on other disciplinary knowledge, as expressed by the proponents of this view, is entirely understandable given nursing's occupational history. The introduction of the Project 2000 reforms of nurse education in the UK, was a decisive move which, for the first time, began to free nursing from the shadows of medicine. Yet whilst released from the dominance of the biomedical paradigm the new broadly based curriculum centred on nursing's 'unique' holistic model, actually contained very little knowledge which was exclusive to nursing. Moreover, with the subject's movement into the higher education sector at a time when many nurse educators lacked an orthodox academic background, there was a real danger that nursing would lose control over its knowledge base as (non-nursing) specialists could teach the nursing curricula. In this context, then, it is understandable why, for certain segments of the nursing research community, the creation of a unique primary nursing discipline is so important.

Nevertheless, a major challenge for those who make the case for independent nursing knowledge is how to define the boundaries of an exclusive discipline. To embark on this course requires some agreement about the boundaries of nursing practice. Even if it were possible to settle upon a definition in a certain historical moment, insights from the sociology of work and occupations would lead us to predict that, in the fullness of time, this would quickly be at odds with daily realities, given the dynamic nature of the world of work which evolves in response to social, economic and political factors (Abbott, 1988). Put slightly differently, what we call 'nursing' does not exist in some essentialist sense, it is a socially constructed concept and claims about what nursing is and its essence have changed in response to changing political and cultural contexts in order to underwrite the occupation's strategies to improve the status, rewards and working conditions of its membership. Furthermore, in different societies the phenomenon 'nursing' is very different (Johnson, 1999). We concur with the views of Johnson.

> [W]e should dispel the notion that there is in some sense a separate epistemology for nursing even it means reminding ourselves that the universe is a big place and has existed for a long time. Our understanding of the physical universe as operating according to 'natural laws' is such that it commits us to the claim that these laws have been in place since the beginning of the universe. The human understanding of these laws is as yet incomplete and crude, with debate about some of the subtleties of method and what counts as a theory worth believing in. Nevertheless, drawing upon positivist methods of data collection and reasoning, 'scientists' working in physical sciences generally have enough confidence in their understanding of these laws to make aeroplanes and most of us have a enough confidence in both the scientists and the manufacturers to fly thousand of miles in them to give papers to academic conferences.
>
> (Johnson, 1999, p. 68)

Indeed, the counter-argument to McKenna and Galvin's (2004) claim that the early nursing scholars who undertook PhDs in related disciplines contributed more to the academic disciplines of sociology and psychology than to nursing per se, is that many of these students *have* made an important contribution to an understanding of nursing *and* cognate fields through the creative insights that arise from combining clinical practitioner knowledge with other disciplinary knowledge. Good examples from the UK might include, Nicky James' work on emotional labour in nursing (1989, 1992b, 1992a, 1993), Clare Williams' (2002) work on mothers, young people and chronic illness which draw on social sciences, and Mandy Fader's work (2004) on the relationship between incontinence products and intersurface pressures which was undertaken in a biomechanics laboratory.

It is possibly its relative immaturity and its power and status vis-à-vis other disciplines that has resulted in such energetic efforts within nursing to create a knowledge base it can call its own. More established applied disciplines seem rather more content to build their knowledge on related primary disciplines. Yet their status may have rather more to do with their historical social power than so-called autonomous bodies of knowledge which serve a largely symbolic purpose (Larson, 1977) and once such status is achieved funding follows which enables the cognitive basis of the discipline to then be developed (Becher, 1989). Established disciplines have no need to justify their existence through reference to an exclusive body of knowledge as their status and worth are secure. Moreover, as disciplinary boundaries throughout the academy are becoming less distinct, it may be the case that in trying to fix its disciplinary basis in too exclusive terms nursing may find itself swimming against the tide of current trends in the evolution of bodies of knowledge. Indeed there are those who work in the interstices of subject areas who have closer affiliations with members of other knowledge communities than they do within their own parent discipline. But what are the prospects for creative synergies between nursing and other knowledge fields? In the next part of this chapter, we consider nursing's relationship with other disciplines, taking sociology and the biomedical sciences as case study examples.

Nursing and sociology

In the UK nursing and sociology have an established association. Nurses are well-represented in the British Sociological Association (BSA) Medical Sociology Group and a number of nurses regularly contribute to the two major UK social science and medicine journals: *Sociology of Health and Illness* and *Social Science and Medicine*. Yet the relationship between the two disciplines is far from harmonious. In 1998, the programme organizers of the BSA annual medical sociology conference created a specific nursing stream, causing considerable disquiet among nurse-sociologists. The latter were aggrieved first, because for them the value of the conference was the interdisciplinarity it afforded and they did not appreciate such segregation and second, because the nursing stream was allocated to a lecture theatre some distance from the heart of the conference, it appeared to accord it a marginal or peripheral status. The reaction of nurse sociologists took the programme organizers by surprise. Faced with the difficult job of organizing the conference programme, the creation of a nursing stream was a rational response to the growing numbers of abstracts submitted on nursing issues and the room allocation had occurred by accident rather than by design. Yet for the nurse-sociologists, the decisions of the programme organizers fed into wider concerns about the relationship between the two disciplines.

In the UK in the 1990s there was a lively debate about the value of sociology's inclusion in the nursing curriculum. The catalyst was an article by Hannah Cooke (1993) which appeared in *Nurse Education Today* which was broadly supportive of the benefits of sociology for nursing but critical of its mode of integration into nurse education. In supporting sociology's incorporation into nursing knowledge, Cooke points to the value of the sociological imagination (Mills, 1970) as a vehicle for encouraging a critical distance from taken-for-granted assumptions and to consider the health care world from a different stance. However, Cooke complains that rather than promoting a more critical perspective, sociology has been appropriated for professional purposes to provide a warrant for the extension of nursing jurisdiction to include the psychosocial as well as the biological functioning of the patient. As a consequence, she argues, nursing curricula have tended to concentrate on the micro social theories of action or at least the micro social consequences of macro processes. What are ignored, Cooke argues, are theories of social structure and those which are critical of nursing work and the institutional contexts in which it takes place.

Cooke's observations can be extended to the research field where, from the diverse range of theoretical frameworks and methodologies available within the sociological tool box, a disproportionate number of nurse researchers have chosen the phenomenological interview. Their efforts to apply this approach to nursing issues have provoked considerable criticism from within the social scientific community. In 1998 writing for *Medical Sociology News*, which is the newsletter of the British Sociological Association Medical Sociology Group, David Hughes reported on the Fourth International Qualitative Health Research (QHR) Conference, Vancouver (Hughes, 1998).

> I detected a perceptible difference between the truly multidisciplinary Hershey conference of 1994 and the two more recent conferences. In Vancouver fewer sociologists were present, nursing emerged as the lead discipline and there seemed to be less theoretical and methodological variety. Put shortly, an awful lot of the papers were based on in-depth interviews, used a version of grounded theory or 'latent content analysis', and sought to delineate the subjective perspectives of carers or sufferers. The success of

the research enterprise was seen to turn largely on the researcher's ability to empathise, to describe, to understand, and only secondarily on the adequacy of analysis of social interaction, social organisation or social structures. Many were less than sophisticated in their conceptualisation of the nature of subjective perspectives and their linkage to action, their selection of data to represent those perspectives, and the analysis of those data. Too many delegates engaged in a certain discourse about qualitative research – emphasising its 'richness', its sensitivity and fidelity to its subjects – which came across as over-romanticised and even maudlin [...] A British delegate said that she found it surprising that basic points covered in any decent social research methods text from 15 years ago were received with adulation as innovative insights. It was difficult to escape the impression that QHR is not just a forum for promoting and disseminating a particular style of research, but also a charismatic social movement.

(Hughes, 1998, p. 21)

Hughes' criticisms of the QHR conference speak to wider emerging criticisms about the over-utilization of the open-ended interview in social sciences in general and in nursing in particular. For example, Atkinson and Silverman (1997) critique the 'romantic impulse' in social science which elevates the experience as authentic and renders the biographical work of interviewer and interviewee invisible. They see this as part of a wider zeitgeist in which the production of selves and lives is accorded special significance. They argue that:

[w]e should not allow a renewed sensitivity to the narrative organization of everyday life to result in an untheorized and uncritical endorsement of personal narratives themselves. They are not, in other words, any more authentic or pure a reflection of the self than any other socially organized set of practices.

(Atkinson and Silverman, 1997, p. 322)

These criticisms are directed explicitly at nursing research by Silverman (1998) in a 'critical but constructive look at current qualitative health research'. He scrutinizes four articles from the journal *Qualitative Health Research* which has a close relationship with the conference considered by Hughes above. The articles, Silverman claims, were selected for convenience in order to develop his arguments, but he is also at pains to point out that the journal editor is a nurse and many of the journal's contributors are in university nursing departments. Having set out his own methodological stall, Silverman finds the articles wanting in a number of respects. The most common criticism is that there is an over-reliance on the open-ended interview and lack of attention to analytic concerns or issues of validity or reliability. He notes that references to grounded theory are commonplace and yet this often seems to serve no other purpose than bestowing scientific legitimacy on the research process. As a consequence categories 'emerge' from the data but it is never entirely clear from whence they have come or by what route. According to Silverman the articles display a lack of analytic nerve which treats research as simply reporting what respondents tell you. Criticizing health researchers for their inability to think theoretically, Silverman asks how understanding a problem from the patients' perspective is real research as opposed to human interest journalism or Oprah Winfrey? He concedes that such theoretical detachment may present particular challenges for health care practitioners. First because their preference for the study of 'people' rather than variables may lead to the pursuit of a kind of 'empathy' which does not permit sufficient distance. Second, in researching an area like health which generates so many pressing social problems, it may sometimes be difficult to look beyond what common-sense knowledge tells you about the 'meaning' of social situations. Nonetheless, he concludes that: 'researchers may have to forego a proportion of their pleasant hot baths in 'empathic' exchanges with interview-respondents and to think critically about the siren-calls of 'humanity' and 'authenticity'.

So what is going on here? Hughes and Silverman are not alone in their publicly expressed concerns about the quality of qualitative research undertaken by members of the health care professions (see also Green, 1998a, 1998b). One might argue, albeit defensively, that this is simply evidence of the 'boundary work' (Gieryn, 1983) of medical sociologists protecting their territory in an area where competition for funds is fierce. As an emergent discipline, nursing must face the competitive demands of more established knowledge communities. Once health professions start appropriating the methods of the social sciences, this may call into question the added value of the social scientist in a research team. It is also the case, however, that qualitative researchers have to compete fiercely in research arena characterized by a hierarchy of research methods, approaches and questions. Given the long and hard fought battle to establish the credibility of these methods in a hostile environment, established researchers are justifiably concerned that what they consider to be poorly executed qualitative work will prove damaging. As we have seen, Gournay's (1999) assessment of the quality of qualitative research undertaken by nurses led him to conclude that nursing research would be better served by a shift to quantitative methodologies.

Whilst these criticisms are well-founded from a social scientific perspective, it is easy to understand why nurse researchers have adopted qualitative research methodologies in the way that they have. Inspired by a particular version of phenomenology which has as its aim the exploration of real world lived experiences, the attraction of the technique for nursing is obvious. A respect for persons and the quality of relationships with clients lies at the heart of nursing's public claims to professional expertise (Aldridge, 1994; Allen, 2001; Salvage, 1992). The roots of this lie in psychodynamic theory in which emphasis is placed on the 'authenticity' of a relationship and the 'uniqueness of individuals'. Yet in practice the social organization of nursing work means that the processes by which nurses interact with patients are neither sustained nor proceed in a linear fashion (May, 1992). Rather nursing work is organized around a fragmented and contingent set of encounters which severely constrains relationship building (see also Latimer, 2000; Allen, 2001). Given its natural affinity with contemporary nursing's jurisdictional claims (see for example Holmes, 1990) and the mismatch between these claims and practice, it is not surprising, that nurse researchers embrace so enthusiastically the open-ended interview as a research method to enable them to develop an understanding of patient experiences which is frequently impossible to achieve in the fast-moving health services world. It is interesting to note the emotional burden described by Lesley Lowes in Chapter 10 of interviewing her own clients and why this should emerge as a feature of the researcher rather than the clinical role. Moreover, the impetus behind much nursing research is to inform practice rather than develop theory. From this perspective, an atheoretical piece of work which has pedagogical utility and provides insights that can be applied to practice has more value than theoretically sophisticated studies that have no pragmatic import. Nevertheless, the real danger, as Hughes notes musing on his Vancouver experience, is that these differences will lead to a parting of the ways and the possibilities for productive engagement between the different communities represented will fail to be realized.

Nursing and the biomedical sciences

In contrast to the social sciences, the involvement of nurses with research based on the biomedical sciences is much more limited. Thompson (2003) points out that few nurses are engaged in clinical science or have been trained in laboratory research. 'This is not to say that all nurses should be laboratory scientists, but it would be nice to have some!' At first sight, this is surprising, given that, for many years, the education of nurses was based on the biomedical paradigm. The reasons for this provide us with further insights into the context of nursing research today.

The term 'medical research' has been used for many years in major documents from the Department of Health to refer to the broad range of inquiry into health service services practice and has been influential in setting the research agenda (Traynor and Rafferty, 1997). This encompasses population-based studies, such as epidemiology, but is most closely associated with the biomedical sciences which form the foundation of clinical practice, such as anatomy, biochemistry, physiology, genetics and pharmacology These disciplines are concerned with describing and understanding the operation of the natural world, including the human body in health and illness and require, for their proper understanding, the ability to comprehend and manipulate concepts derived from the fundamental sciences: mathematics, physics, chemistry and biology.

In Chapter 10 of this book, Weeks describes his early studies which were initiated by his experience, as a nurse lecturer, observing the difficulties experienced by students who were trying to grasp simple mathematical principles. Such difficulties are very common in students from many areas. Like mathematics, biological science has, for many years, been seen as a cause of student difficulty and stress (Akinsanya, 1984; Sutcliffe, 1992). It is not, therefore surprising that few nurses are naturally drawn to these subjects, although many do develop a satisfactory working knowledge of the biological sciences required by their practice, particularly in the more specialized areas. However, in order to function as a researcher in these disciplines, a thorough grounding in both them and their underlying sciences is required and this is difficult to achieve without firm early foundations. Therefore, while nurses may indeed become familiar with and proficient in the biosciences at an applied level, it is rare for those who have not undergone the normal educational preparation of a scientist to reach the level required in order to become a scientific researcher.

Lack of opportunity and adverse early experiences are two reasons for the limited engagement of nurses with bioscience research. There is the possibility that the 'non-intuitive' nature of science described below is another. Finally, the perception in some quarters that the adoption of a scientific approach is at odds with caring might also be a contributory factor. By its very nature, research in the natural sciences requires detachment from human factors. This has produced what some term a 'dualism' between the natural sciences and the human science paradigm which has become prominent in nurse education, particularly in North America (Chan, 2002). Unfortunately some nurse scholars make the assumption that adopting a detached stance when engaged in scientific work implies a general world view that is opposed to the holistic nature of caring. This tends to give all science a bad image and implies that any scientist lacks concern for the 'whole person' in all fields of activity. Terms such as 'hard', 'reductionist' and 'positivistic', are sometimes applied in a derogatory sense, to work of this kind, although scientists themselves use them as positive adjectives to describe their science.

The emergence of the biomedical sciences as we know them today has been accompanied by an evolving relationship between practical and theoretical developments. Some commentators see this in terms of interactions between those who have made practical improvements through experience (the technologists), those who have reasoned on the basis of theory (the scientists) and those who have provided practical assistance to both (the technicians). For example, Wolpert (1992) views technology as atheoretical and concerned with the production of useful artefacts (or processes) through practical experience. Technology was responsible for most developments which have benefited humanity up to the mid-nineteenth century. Only in the last 200 years has science come to the aid of technology and enabled the spectacular progress of modern times. According to Wolpert, science is distinguished from technology by being concerned with how the natural world works (rather than 'what works'). It is theoretically based and describable in mathematical language. Whilst technology advanced from the time of early man to the present day, science 'happened' for the first time in Greece, around 600 BC, when Thales of Miletos attempted to derive general principles governing the natural world without any reference to man's relation to it. Although technology later influenced science, by providing tools and techniques to investigate natural phenomena, the converse was not true until 200 years ago.

Wolpert's is perhaps an extreme view of the distinction between science and technology and is more subtle than the above brief outline indicates. However, he makes a suggestion which is of particular relevance to the relationship between nursing research and the natural sciences. He demonstrates that science is often counter-intuitive and proposes that the human brain has evolved in response to practical problems in the environment, resulting in 'common sense' as a dominant form of thought leading to technological progress. The counter-intuitive nature of science is one of the main reasons for scientists seeking to maintain their distance from human perceptual factors in the conduct of their research, since those things that we intuitively 'know' to be true (i.e. which are common sense) are constantly open to challenge in the natural world. Of course social and other factors come into play in the lives of scientists, the choices they make and the way they communicate with the wider world (Gilbert and Mulkay, 1984; Callon *et al.*, 1988) and these have been emphasized by critics who decry notions of scientific objectivity. However, this misunderstands the absolute requirement for the science to be uncontaminated in order to allow the counter-intuitive to be perceived.

Common sense is a quality which is highly and rightly valued in nursing. But it has its limitations, notably the way that it restricts our ability to understand that which is true but counter-intuitive. Take a very simple example. When presented with some data which shows the intersurface pressure between a seated person and the substrate, most nursing students are reluctant at first to believe that these pressures are lower in heavy people than in light ones. Common sense dictates that the heavier person is at greater risk of tissue damage. Science explains that body configuration is more important than weight in determining the intersurface pressure, so that in a light person with protuberant bones all the force is concentrated on a small area. In nursing practice, many common sense procedures (e.g. tipping the head of the bed when the patient becomes hypotensive) have been shown to be inappropriate by the underlying physiology.

In the past, technological, common sense thinking has led to major developments in, for example, agriculture, engineering, public health and transport. Wolpert's suggestion that the human brain has evolved in response to the success of this type of thinking has no empirical support, but, if true, could explain why this is the dominant mode of thought today. In contrast, the propensity for scientific thought might be seen as a less common attribute, like, for example, musical or artistic ability, having been much less useful in evolutionary terms. Whilst creative abilities are acknowledged to be scarce and are highly esteemed in society, scientific ability is not very well appreciated outside the scientific community.

For the most part, the involvement of nurses with medical and biomedical research has been largely as technicians, i.e. as data collectors supporting medical studies or performing routine tests. Over time, this role has evolved to that of the trial coordinator, a highly skilled function, drawing on nursing knowledge, which has almost assumed the status of a technology in its own right (Nelson *et al.*, 2003). However it is true to say that while the trialists may develop methodological expertise in trial design and sampling, they are not expected to investigate the mode of action of drugs or the reasons for the efficacy of interventions, i.e. they are not expected to engage with the underlying science and therefore scientific ability and training are not a requirement.

In areas of care that have been long recognized as primary nursing functions, a different situation has developed. Here, nurses have undertaken technological studies, at first in collaboration with technologists (Bowker and Davidson, 1979), then in their own right and have lately become more interested in the science and begun to address the theoretical questions underlying areas such as continence promotion, nutrition, infection control, tissue viability, pain and stress.

Take tissue viability as an example. This covers issues around the promotion of skin integrity, and the healing of wounds. Early studies by nurses concentrated on pressure ulcers (PU) and were descriptive, leading to estimates of the incidence of this condition and the identification of risk factors (Norton, 1996; Waterlow, 1988), with the nurses acting in a technical capacity to locate and describe PU where they occurred. However, the need to produce improved methods of risk assessment led first to technological advance and then to the involvement of nurses who had developed expertise in the underlying mathematical disciplines and were able to adopt a theoretically informed approach to the whole question of risk assessment (Anthony *et al.*, 2000). In parallel with these moves came a similar progression in the area of skin integrity and wound healing. Initially the involvement of nurses was confined to the technical aspects of trials of dressings and appliances, to determine 'what works' and this line of enquiry has continued with good effect up to the present day, with nurses taking a more prominent role in the management of such studies (Macauley *et al.*, 2004). Gradually their involvement has widened and nurses with an interest in this area have pioneered methodological advances (Browne *et al.*, 2003), improved research designs (Nelson *et al.*, 2003; Nixon *et al.*, 2000) and moved into the laboratory to study the underlying science in order to improve understanding of the physiology of wound healing (Voegeli *et al.*, 1999).

This progression mirrors the move from technology to science which Wolpert describes. It seems to have occurred in areas of study which were not previously fully colonized by biomedical scientists. In order to function as scientists within these fields, however, nurses have been obliged to become properly trained in the biosciences; a nursing qualification is not an adequate preparation for high quality laboratory based science. As we have seen, critics suggest that work of this nature can no longer be regarded as 'nursing' (Fawcett, 2003; RCN, 2004). The counter-argument is that the nurse with expertise in biotechnology or bioscience can ensure that important gaps in the knowledge needed to advance practice are addressed and can contribute to the development of bioscience theory which is needed to underpin practice and bridge the gulf between nursing practice and laboratory science.

Where nurses do operate in this environment they are acknowledged as bioscientists by their peers as long as they have the right credentials. The objectivity of science, which is sometimes questioned or even derided by nurse scholars is an advantage here because the quality of published or examined work, in terms of generally agreed criteria, is relatively easy to demonstrate and the work can be tested by replication. Nurse scientists do not form a recognisable sub-group, unlike the nurse social scientists described above and there is no record of a comparable interaction between nurse bioscientists and their colleagues. The only circumstance in which a comparable situation might exist would be where nurses were using the results of their bioscience research in order to investigate an issue which created tension between them and colleagues, for example, in investigating a postulated gendered aspect of medical practice or questioning some reconfiguration of service provision. Under these circumstances, criticism might be levelled on the grounds that the work was of poor quality, but these could easily be refuted. More likely would be criticism of the interpretation of the findings. This will become a challenge in the future if the involvement of nurses in scientific research extends further from the areas of traditional nursing jurisdiction. Thompson (2003) points to the increasing number of nurses taking leadership roles in research which draws on the biosicences, for example in specialized areas such as cardiovascular nursing. It is in such circumstances that the politics of health care could impact upon the acceptance of the outputs of laboratory based research produced by nurses.

Interdisciplinary, multidisciplinary and transdisciplinary research

Bushaway (2003) argues that university-based research has evolved towards increasing specialization on a relatively narrow basis. Attempts have been made to counter this tendency through the creation of horizontal structures which bring together researchers from different disciplines. In the 1980s in the UK the research councils funded the establishment of centres of excellence to foster interdisciplinary research and multidisciplinary teams are becoming an important feature in the research landscape as research funding becomes more selectively allocated to expert teams tackling big problems. Increasingly, applicants for research funding are required to articulate explicitly why the proposed team is well-placed to undertake the work.

Those who consider it to be perfectly legitimate for nursing research to look to the insights of related disciplinary fields, often point to the value of collaboration with members of more established disciplines as a useful strategy in developing nursing research capacity and providing an entrée to key funding bodies (Gournay and Ritter, 1997). Lindsay et al. (2001) analyse the characteristics of research outputs from the top three rated nursing departments in the 1996 RAE in order to identify 'gold standard' characteristics for research papers. The authors are not concerned with 'quality' per se, rather their focus is what they call 'context characteristics': publication source, characteristics of authors (numbers, location by institution and discipline), the funding sources, classification of subject matter. They found that papers written in collaboration with others are more likely to be externally funded and papers written in collaboration with other disciplines are more likely to be funded than those written jointly by nurses.

Yet nursing suffers from a lack of academic credibility in the eyes of other disciplines (Traynor and Rafferty, 1998) which can make establishing collaborative partnerships difficult. In the competitive environment of higher education in which RAE scores translate into funding decisions, established departments have little incentive to engage in partnership working with weaker players and, indeed, some universities' institutional policies may expressly discourage this. Another challenge is that, in the field of multidisciplinary health services research, the hierarchical relationships which characterize the clinical field get mapped onto the research relationship, with the result that the multidisciplinary working can be a mixed blessing. Whilst it has encouraged doctors to seek research partners from other professional research groups, it has been difficult for all but a small number of nurses to participate as equals with doctors on multi-disciplinary teams. Lorentzon (1995) argues that the skills of the therapy professions are specific and necessary in healthcare and there is little risk of their being taken over by other professionals, but the different position occupied by the generic nursing profession which makes nursing flexible and open to new developments, also leaves it vulnerable in the R&D context. Luker (1999) observes, that many nurses who have made such a transition are reluctant to acclaim their nursing origins: most consider themselves to be rebadged to as, for example, social scientist or epidemiologist. Luker argues that: 'this is fine for the mainstream NHS research and development agenda, but it means that nursing as a discipline struggles to recruit able research staff, and the nursing component of the National R&D agenda remains rather under-powered'.

Conclusion

In this chapter we have examined the field of nursing research. We have considered the breadth and diversity of nursing research concerns and have explored methodological debates within this segmented community of knowledge. Nursing's relationships with other disciplines have been examined and consideration given to the implications these have for the discipline in a climate in which there is a growing tendency for research to be multidisciplinary. During the process of writing this chapter we are drawn to the inescapable conclusion that the involvement of nurses in multidisciplinary teams is either as a representative of professional nursing or as a researcher with expertise in a parent discipline, either social or biomedical science. It is our experience that other disciplines will respect expertise whenever they encounter it and will allow that a nurse can have such expertise. Medical colleagues, for example, will acknowledge that they do not have qualitative expertise and some are willing to concede that it is a specialism and respect it as such. However, it seems that nursing is not seen as a specialism of the same calibre. The challenge for nursing is to consider whether it can resolve these dilemmas concerning the status of nursing as a research discipline with its own sphere of knowledge or repertoire of techniques, or should it grasp the nettle and admit that it is not, but that it is one of many disciplines which synthesizes and applies knowledge and skills derived from other disciplines to a field of study which is defined and informed by professional insight. This is exactly the same situation in medicine, so why should we worry?

Acknowledgements

This chapter draws on a previously published manuscript: Allen, D. (2001) Review Article: The marriage of nursing and sociology: An uneasy relationship? *Sociology of Health and Illness* 23 (3): 386–96, which is reproduced with permission from Blackwell Publishing.

References

Abbott, A. (1988) *The System of Professions: An Essay on the Division of Expert Labor*, Chicago: University of Chicago Press.

Akinsanya, J. (1984) 'Development of a nursing knowledge base in the life sciences: problems and prospects', *International Journal of Nursing Studies*, 21, 221–7.

Aldridge, M. (1994) 'Unlimited liability? Emotional labour in nursing and social work', *Journal of Advanced Nursing*, 20, 722–8.

Allen, D. (2001) *The Changing Shape of Nursing Practice: The Role of Nurses in the Hospital Division of Labour*, London: Routledge.

—— (2004) 'Ethnomethodological insights into insider-outsider relationships in nursing ethnographies of healthcare settings', *Nursing Inquiry*, 11, 14–24.

Anthony, D., Clark, M. and Dallender, J. (2000) 'An optimisation of the Waterlow score using regression and artificial neural networks', *Clinical Rehabilitation*, 14, 102–9.

Atkinson, P. and Silverman, D. (1997) 'Kundera's *Immortality*: the interview society and the invention of the self', *Qualitative Inquiry*, 3, 304–25.

Becher, T. (1989) *Academic Tribes and Territories: Intellectual Enquiry and the Cultures of Disciplines*, Milton Keynes: Open University Press.

Bond, S. (2002) *UOA10 – Nursing. Overall Assessment of the Sector*, London: HERO.

Bowker, P. and Davidson, L.M. (1979) 'Development of a cushion to prevent ischial pressure sores', *British Medical Journal*, 2, 958–61.

Browne, N., Grocutt, P., Cowley, S., Cameron, J., Dealey, C., Keogh, A., Lovatt A., Vowden, K. and Vowden, P. (2003) 'Wound care research for appropriate products (WRAP): validation of the TELER method involving users', *International Journal of Nursing Studies*, 41, 559–71.

Bulmer, M. (1987) *Social Science Research and the Government: Comparative Essays on Britain and the United States*, Cambridge: Cambridge University Press.

Bushaway, R.W. (2003) *Managing Research*, Maidenhead: Open University Press.

Callon, M., Law, J. and Rip, A. (eds) (1988) *Mapping the Dynamics of Science and Technology*, Basingstoke: Macmillan.

Carter-Snell, C. and Hegadoren, K. (2003) 'Stress disorders and gender: implications for theory and research', *Canadian Journal of Nursing Research*, 35, 34–55.

Chan, E.A. (2002) 'A lived experience of dualism between the natural and human science paradigms in nursing', *Journal of Advanced Nursing*, 40, 739–46.

Charles, C. (1988) *Introduction to Educational Research*, New York: Longman.

Cooke, H. (1993) 'Why teach sociology?', *Nurse Education Today*, 13, 210–16.

Craig, G. (1997) *Quality First? The Assessment of Quality in Social Policy Research*, London: Social Policy Association.

Cutcliffe, J.R. and Goward, P. (2000) 'Mental health nurses and qualitative research methods: a mutual attraction?', *Journal of Advanced Nursing*, 31, 590–8.

De Waal Malefit, A. (1974) *Images of Man: A History of Anthropological Thought*, New York: Knopf.

Eagleton, T. (1983) *Literary Theory: An Introduction*, Oxford: Blackwell.

Fader, M., Bain, D. and Cottenden, A. (2004) 'Effects of adsorbent incontinence pads on pressure management mattresses', *Journal of Advanced Nursing*, 48, 569–74.

Fawcett, J. (2000a) *Analysis and Evaluation of Contemporary Nursing Knowledge: Nursing Models and Theories*, Philadelphia, PA: F. A. Davies.

—— (2000b) 'The state of nursing science: where is the nursing in the science?', *Theoria: Journal of Nursing Theory*, 9, 3–10.

—— (2003) Guest editorial: 'On bed baths and conceptual models of nursing', *Journal of Advanced Nursing*, 44, 229–30.

Gieryn, T. (1983) 'Boundary-work and the demarcation of science from non-science: strains and interests in professional ideologies of scientists', *American Sociological Review*, 48, 781–95.

Gilbert, N.G. and Mulkay, M. (1984) *Opening Pandora's Box: A Sociological Analysis of Scientists' Discourse*, Cambridge: Cambridge University Press.

Gournay, K. (1999) 'The future of nursing research will be better served by a shift to quantitative methodologies', *Clinical Effectiveness in Nursing*, 3, 1–3.

Gournay, K. and Ritter, S. (1997) 'What future for research in mental health nursing', *Journal of Psychiatric and Mental Health Nursing*, 4, 441–6.

Graeff, G. (1987) *Professing Literature: An Institutional History*, Chicago: University of Chicago Press.

Green, J. (1998a) 'Commentary: grounded theory and the constant comparative method', *British Medical Journal*, 316, 1064–5.

—— (1998b) *Doing Health Services Research*, York: British Sociological Association Medical Sociology Group Annual Conference.

Hirst, P. (1975) 'The nature and structure of curriculum objectives', in M. Golby, J. Greenwald and R. West (eds) *Curriculum Design*, Beckenham: Croom Helm.

Holmes, C.A. (1990) 'Alternatives to natural science foundations for nursing', *International Journal of Nursing Studies*, 27, 187–98.

Hughes, D. (1998) The Fourth International Qualitative Health Research Conference, Vancouver, 19–21 February 1998, *Medical Sociology News*, 24, 20–2.

James, N. (1989) 'Emotional labour: skill and work in the social regulation of feelings', *The Sociological Review*, 37, 15–41.

—— (1992a) 'Care = organisation + physical labour = emotional labour', *Sociology of Health and Illness*, 14, 488–509.

—— (1992b) 'Care, work and carework: a synthesis?', in J. Robinson, A. Gray and R. Elkan (eds) *Policy Issues in Nursing*, Milton Keynes: Open University Press.

—— (1993) 'Divisions of emotional labour: Disclosure and cancer', in Fineman, S. (ed.) *Emotion in Organizations*. London, Sage Publications.

Johnson, M. (1999) 'Observations on positivism and pseudoscience in qualitative nursing research', *Journal of Advanced Nursing*, 30, 67–73.

Johnson, M., Long, T. and While, A. (2001) 'Arguments for "British Pluralism" in qualitative health research', *Journal of Advanced Nursing*, 33, 243–9.

Larson, M.S. (1977) *The Rise of Professionalism: A Sociological Analysis*, Berkley, CA: University of California Press.

Latimer, J. (2000) *The Conduct of Care: Understanding Nursing Practice*, Oxford: Blackwell Science.

Lawton, J. (2000) *The Dying Process: Patients' Experiences of Palliative Care*, London: Routledge.

Lindsay, B., Macdonald, H. and Cooper, N. (2001) *Assessing the Characteristics of Nursing Research Publications: The Nursing and Midwifery Output Study*, Norwich,:Nursing and Midwifery Research Unit, University of East Anglia.

Lorentzon, M. (1995) Guest editorial: 'Multidisciplinary collaboration: Lifeline or drowning pool for nurse researchers?', *Journal of Advanced Nursing*, 22, 825–6.

Luker, K.A. (1999) 'The dilemma concerning the nurse's role in a multidisciplinary research agenda', *Nursing Times Research*, 4, 85–6.

Macauley, M., Petterson, L., Fader, M., Cottenden, A. and Brooks, R. (2004) 'Disposable pull-ups versus disposable nappies for children with a disability', *Nursing Times*, 100, 64–5.

May, C. (1992) 'Nursing work, nurses' knowledge, and the subjectification of the patient', *Sociology of Health and Illness*, 14, 472–87.

McKenna, H. and Galvin, K. (2004) 'Doctoral processes: the scholarly practitioner', in D. Freshwater and V. Bishop (eds) *Nursing Research in Context: Appreciation, Applications and Professional Developments*, Basingstoke: Palgrave Macmillan.

Mills, C.W. (1970) *The Sociological Imagination*, London: Pelican.

Monaghan, L. (2001) 'Looking good, feeling good: the embodied pleasures of vibrant physicality', *Sociology of Health and Illness*, 23, 330–56.

Mulholland, J. (1997) 'Assimilating sociology: critical reflections on the "Sociology in nursing" debate', *Journal of Advanced Nursing*, 25, 844–52.

Nelson, E.A., Nixon, J., Mason, S., Barrow, H., Phillips, A. and Cullum, N. (2003) 'A nurse led randomised trial of pressure relieving support surfaces', *Professional Nurse*, 18, 513–16.

Nixon, J., Brown, J., McElvenny, D., Bainbridge, J. and Mason, S. (2000) 'Some practical issues in the design, monitoring and analysis of sequential randomized trial in pressure sore prevention', *Statistics in Medicine*, 19, 3389–400.

Norton, D. (1996) 'Calculating the risk: reflections on the Norton Scale', *Advances in Wound Care*, 9, 38–43.

Parse, R.R. (1981) *Man-Living-Health: A Theory of Nursing*, New York: Wiley.

—— (2000) 'Paradigms: a reprise', *Nursing Science Quarterly*, 12, 275.

Rafferty, A.M. (1995) *Political Leadership in Nursing*, Final Harkness Fellowship Report, Commonwealth Fund of New York.

Ray, L. (1999) 'Evidence and outcomes: agendas, presuppositions and power', *Journal of Advanced Nursing*, 30, 1017–26.

RCN (2004) *Research Ethics*, London, RCN.

Rogers, M.E. (1980) *An Introduction to the Theoretical Basis of Nursing*, Philadelphia, PA: Davies.

—— (1992) 'Nursing science and the space age', *Nursing Science Quarterly*, 7, 33–5.

Rolfe, G. (1997) 'Knowledge, power and authority: a response to Gournay and Ritter', *Journal of Psychiatric and Mental Health Nursing*, 4, 441–6.

Salvage, J. (1992) 'The new nursing: empowering patients or empowering nurses?', in J. Robinson, A. Gray and R. Elkan (eds) *Policy Issues in Nursing*, Milton Keynes: Open University Press.

Silverman, D. (1998) 'The quality of qualitative health research: the open-ended interview and its alternatives', *Social Sciences in Health*, 4, 104–18.

Solanti, H. (2002) 'Midwifery research: the past, the present and future', *Midwives*, 5, 384–6.

Sutcliffe, L. (1992) 'An investigation into whether nurses change their learning styles according to subject area studied', *Journal of Advanced Nursing*, 18, 647–58

Thompson, D.R. (2003) Editorial: 'Thinking bigger about research', *Journal of Advanced Nursing*, 43, 1–2

Traynor, M. and Rafferty, A.M. (1997) *The NHS R&D Context for Nursing Research: A Working Paper*, London: Centre for Policy in Nursing Research, London School of Hygiene and Tropical Medicine.

—— (1998) *Nursing Research and the Higher Education Context: A Second Working Paper*, London: Centre for Policy in Nursing Research, London School of Hygiene and Tropical Medicine.

Traynor, M., Rafferty, A. and Lewinson, G. (2001) 'Endogenous and exogenous research? Findings from a bibliometric study of UK nursing research', *Journal of Advanced Nursing*, 34, 212–22.

Voegeli, D., Clough, G.F. and Church, M.K. (1999) 'Localisation of microdialysis probes in human skin in vivo', *Journal of Vascular Research*, 36, 334.

Waterlow, J. (1988) 'The Waterlow card for the prevention and management of pressure sores: towards a pocket policy', *Care: Science and Practice*, 6, 8–12.

Watkin, D. (1980) *The Rise of Architectural History*, Chicago, IL: The University of Chicago Press.

Williams, C. (2002) *Mothers, Young People and Chronic Illness*, Aldershot: Ashgate.

Wolpert, L. (1992) *The Unnatural Nature of Science*, London: Faber and Faber.

Chapter 5

The continuum of research engagement

Davina Allen and Patricia Lyne

Introduction

The Briggs Report called for nursing to be a research-based profession, recognizing that the 'sense of the need for research should become part of the mental equipment of every practising nurse or midwife' (Traynor and Rafferty, 1998). It is now widely accepted that research is every nurse, midwife or health visitor's business, but 30 years after *Briggs* the precise meaning and implications of this statement have rarely been considered in full. There is a lack of specificity concerning the function of research in the diverse roles nurses occupy and the skills needed to perform at any particular level. This lack of clarity is evident in many of the documents which set out national policies for the development of nursing research and the literature on evidence-based practice. It arises from several unresolved issues, for example the inherent tensions between professional and managerial versions of EBP and the varied expectations of the products of research. The appropriate focus for 'nursing' research is still debated, with authors such as Fawcett (2003) rejecting as unsuitable for nurse researchers the investigation of any phenomenon which does not have its roots in a conceptual model of nursing. It is also true that the relationship between research-based and other forms of evidence to support nursing practice remains contentious. Given all these major debates, it is not surprising that few authors have looked past them to consider how nurses, in their various and varied roles, actually engage with research, or to put it another way, what modes of engagement with research are demanded by these roles and how might nurses be prepared in each case. Equally important is a consideration of what is not required or expected of a given role.

Towards a typology of modes of engagement

As these debates continue, it is clear that nurses in clinical and educational settings are engaging with research in different ways and at different levels according to their particular role. For example, a nurse researcher undertaking original research is doing something quite different from a nurse manager with responsibility for implementing evidence in clinical practice and the two require different skill sets. So a variety of modes of engagement exist and in this chapter we will describe the progress that has been made towards making their distinct and varied nature more visible.

An early attempt to capture this diversity was made in 1982 by Shirley Stinson and colleagues in Canada, who listed a total of 18 examples of 'staff nurse roles in nursing research' (Stinson, 2004). These included the traditional such as investigator, critiquer, organizer, interpreter and also the less obvious such as doubter, philosopher and even fund raiser. In Europe, ways of engaging with research have been defined in broader terms. For example, Freshwater and Bishop (2003), writing specifically about research based in clinical practice, describe three levels of involvement: a general level (conducting evidence-based practice and assessing the quality of research); a facilitative level (encouraging and supporting researchers) and a personal level (conducting research). The need to progress further was identified by researchers in the School of Nursing and Midwifery, Cardiff University, whose work informed the development of a strategy for Nursing, Midwifery and Health Visiting in Wales, introducing a sense of the dynamic nature of research engagement throughout the career: 'A continuum of engagement (with research) exists and the individual will work at different points upon it as their career develops' (WAG, 2004).

The Cardiff group (Allen *et al.*, 2004) sought increased clarity about the type and level of engagement with research required by individual nursing roles. The initial objective was to develop a framework of modes of research engagement which would support local research capacity building within the School. After health service colleagues also expressed enthusiasm for the proposal, it was extended to include research roles in all the settings in which nurses practise. The starting point was a series of workshops held on the School's Annual Research Day. Participants were requested to bring with them an object which signified their engagement with research and explain the reason for their choices. The feedback from workshop facilitators and subsequent discussion provided the stimulus for the thinking on which the Cardiff Framework of Research Engagement (CFRE) is based. CFRE was produced by a working group with representation from education and practice contexts. It identified and defined nine modes of engagement: producer, utilizer, teacher, supervisor, leader, manager, implementer, influencer and evaluator. Within each mode, several levels were described, forming a progression of expertise. CFRE is currently undergoing evaluation. The following sections draw on the early work, using the modes to illustrate further how the interactions between various influences and discourses, which form a major theme of this book, influence the nature of research in nursing today.

Research utilizer

CFRE defines a research utilizer as 'One who makes use of primary or secondary research directly or indirectly'. This is perhaps the most fundamental and generally accepted mode of engagement with research for nurses and, on the face of it, should be the least contentious. It turns out that the reverse is the case and a detailed exploration of what it might mean to be a research utilizer provides a very good example of the effect of the unresolved issues to which we referred earlier.

There have been many investigations of 'research utilization' which have identified both facilitators and barriers (for example, Funk *et al.*, 1995; Marsh *et al.*, 2001). However, in most cases there is a tacit acceptance that 'utilization' is a single activity and its many facets have not been explored. In order to bring some clarity into the area, we start by reflecting on an important but often overlooked distinction between research as an activity and the various products of that activity (findings, results, evidence, techniques, instruments, processes, artefacts, ideas, insights, etc.). Since the products are diverse, it follows that there is a variety of ways of being a utilizer either directly or indirectly, i.e. after the products have been further processed in some way.

All practitioners make use of interventions and technologies in their daily work, thus directly utilizing the products of research. They are guided by evidence-based guidelines, pathways and protocols; an indirect use of research products after they have been processed by others. They use research literature for personal scholarship. In these cases the situation is relatively straightforward and the skills required of the utilizer are to operate the technologies, apply the guidance and locate the literature, processes which are clearly envisaged in their educational preparation. This might be regarded as the baseline level of research utilization. If so, rather than asserting that research is every nurse's business, it is more appropriate to say that 'The products (or outputs) of research are, in some way or other, every nurse's business'.

Once we move beyond this baseline we reach a more complex situation. In the majority of clinical and managerial situations there is an expectation that the individual will engage in EBP by the direct or indirect use of research findings to inform professional decisions. This is perhaps what most people mean today when they speak of research utilization. In nursing, the professional model of EBP carries the expectation that practitioners will consider a range of factors in addition to research based evidence, to determine best practice for the individual or the group. Di Censo et al. (1998) define evidence-based nursing as the process of decision making which uses the best available research evidence, clinical expertise and patient preferences, together with consideration of the available resources. This definition implies that, when making a clinical decision concerning a group or an individual patient/client, the practitioner will consider and give appropriate weight to information from several sources, including research based guidance. This is much easier to advocate than to do. Ryecroft-Malone et al. (2004) have moved the debate forward by stressing the need to ensure that all types of evidence, including information from experience, the patient and the context, are 'as robust as possible and that they are melded coherently and sensibly in the real time of practice'. They are currently working to develop strategies to support this activity.

The actual demands of synthesizing research-based evidence with information from a range of sources have, in our view, been underestimated. The nature of this challenge is indicated by studies designed to capture the process and produce decision support systems (O'Neill et al., 2004). One reason for this underestimate is to be found in the debate about the 'truth' of research findings. Ryecroft Malone et al. (2004) consider that research evidence is rarely definitive and should be regarded as provisional rather than providing absolute answers to the questions posed. This is perhaps a somewhat partial view of research evidence in that it fails to show that rather than being indefinite, research evidence, properly interpreted, can provide a known degree of uncertainty, which is not the same thing as being provisional. The essence of science (in the very broadest sense) is that it provides answers that have in-built uncertainty. The better the science, the more fully the degree of uncertainty is understood. So statisticians commonly speak of 'the true but unknown value', which is estimated as lying within a defined confidence interval and the Nobel Laureate Richard Feynman argued that 'In physics, the truth is rarely perfectly clear and that is certainly universally the case in human affairs. Hence, whatever is not surrounded by uncertainty cannot be the truth' (Feynman, 2005). This sounds as if, rather than giving a definitive answer, science is asking us to search for a needle in the proverbial haystack. On the contrary, good science will tell us which haystack to look in and the size of the haystack in which the needle of truth is buried. This is worth knowing, because it tells us something definite.

Understanding the degree of uncertainty in research findings is the result of skilful interpretation of those findings and it is essential if they are to be synthesized with others and additional types of information. Although we have used examples from the natural sciences above, the same can be said of any research tradition, including those in which uncertainty is not expressed in mathematical terms. A single case study allows us to make certain statements about the individual with a high degree of certainty. The uncertainty arises in respect of the relationship between that case and other individuals. Such interpretations can only be made from the basis of a firm grasp of the underlying discipline.

Nurses attempting to engage in EBP as individuals have to do even more than appreciate the degree of uncertainty inherent in the relevant primary research or in the available guidance produced by those who have synthesized the evidence. They also need to weigh this against other evidence, from practical experience or patient preferences, of which the degree of uncertainty is completely unknown. This being the case, a fundamental but under-emphasized skill required to engage with research at this level is the ability to understand and balance competing uncertainties of different degrees of precision. Expressed in this way, the magnitude of the task is starkly revealed and places a big question mark against the notion that this type of research utilization can be everybody's business. Conversely, where this expectation does exist in respect of a given nursing role, it is logical to stipulate that the post holder possesses, acquires or has access to the necessary skills and resources. This, it might be said, is certainly every organization's business.

However, the onus is sometimes placed on the individual practitioner. For example, as a result of their study of research utilization by breast care specialist nurses (BCNs), Kirshbaum et al. (2004) found that the highest ranked barrier to research utilization in this group of specialists was 'statistical analysis not understandable' (identified as a great or moderate barrier by 72.6 per cent of respondents). They conclude that it is the responsibility of the individual BCN to remove this barrier by addressing weaknesses in their own understanding of research and statistics, with support from managers and colleagues. One wonders how realistic this aspiration can be. Do the job descriptions of the BCNs require them to engage with research at this level and integrate all forms of evidence in the way that we have described? And if so, what educational level is appropriate for the role?

Others place more emphasis on the role of the organization. The Foundation of Nursing Studies (FoNS) (2001) conclude that rather than through individual action, EBP will better be achieved through the application of care pathways, guidelines and protocols within the organization. The use of research findings in the production of guidance and policy represents a further level of engagement in this mode. It is here that skills in the interpretation of research and the synthesis of evidence (or access to such skills) are essential, together with the managerial capacity to create the conditions in which individual practitioners can be assured that their practice is evidence based and have the freedom to apply their legitimate knowledge and expertise in an appropriate manner. Nurses working at this level may be part of local guideline development teams, clinical governance facilitators or have an organizational remit for R&D. With increasing expertise they undertake systematic reviews and meta analyses, perhaps contributing to national policies, service frameworks and protocols or, in the educational sector, to inform curriculum development and educational policy.

Consideration of this aspect of research utilization, i.e. the use of research findings to inform practice, illustrates what we mean by a continuum of engagement. It brings to light the different levels of expertise and experience required within the utilizer community. In our view, the failure to recognize the full extent of these differences is a real barrier to the advancement of research in nursing. At one end of the research user continuum is the new practitioner who follows evidence-based protocols and thus makes use of existing research indirectly. In order to function within their role, this person does not need to understand competing methodologies and research philosophies, to counterpose relative uncertainties or to have critical appraisal skills. As the practitioner gains experience, he or she is expected to apply problem-solving skills to new questions and interpret research findings in the light of increasing experience. However, he/she will have been prepared to degree or diploma level by an educational programme which contains a research component as a very minor element in a broad-based curriculum. Further along the continuum is the nurse consultant, having research and development as one element in a highly complex role and being expected to act as the bridge spanning research and practice. Even if educated to doctoral level it is unlikely that the nurse consultant will have had the opportunity to become experienced in evidence synthesis, because of the necessity to gain high level clinical, managerial and educational prowess as well. So at both ends of the spectrum there can be a mismatch between the level of preparation and experience and the expectation of the degree of research engagement. This view does not in any way diminish the skills possessed by such practitioners. It merely reinforces the unrealistic nature of the expectations about this type of research utilization placed on people who are developing or have developed expertise on a very wide front. One reason for this, in our view, is that the utilization of research is sometimes seen as a single skill which can be developed along the 'novice to expert' trajectory which is used to describe other important skills in the nursing repertoire. Parahoo (1997) refers to the need for nurses to 'read basic research articles and reports critically and to have a basic understanding of the research process'. The logical extension of this idea is that there is 'simple' research, which can be appreciated by those with a beginning level of understanding and used meaningfully to inform decision-making.

Obviously, some types of research are more accessible than others, and those which use mathematical language are, by their very nature, opaque to the majority of the population who do not speak this language, so that qualitative studies are sometimes seen as being more 'basic' than those which employ quantitative methods. In our view, nothing could be further from the truth and, with very few exceptions, research that has something useful to say is far from 'basic'. Conversely, research that can be regarded as basic in the sense of being easy for anyone to understand fails to convey any sense of the degree of uncertainty of the findings. It contributes to the layer of evidence which is usually termed 'professional opinion'.

In this section we have discussed two aspects of research utilization by nurses, the use of research products in practice and the direct or indirect use of research findings to inform practice. There are others, for example as educationalist using research to inform teaching and as scholar using research to inspire, inform and shape new programmes of work. The important but less tangible function of creating a research culture has been envisioned by several writers, particularly with reference to education. HEFCE (2001) cites a review of research policy by JM Consulting which concluded that the benefits of research for teaching are real and varied but are not necessarily seen at the level of the individual. Rather they accrue through the shared intellectual culture of a department, university or network. The difficulty of achieving such a culture in a nursing faculty was described by Gething *et al.* (2000) who observed that members of the more established faculties in the university could not appreciate the immense effort needed to start from scratch, since it was so natural to them. They were 'steeped in a research culture from early graduate years'.

This notion of the research utilizer, as an informed individual, contributing to the organization's research culture places that function in a network of research engagement which includes production, dissemination and implementation. The importance of this function and the preparation required to perform it have been largely overlooked in the debates about research in nurse education, which appear to have focused on the conduct of research by academics. It might be suggested that enhancing skills in the utilization of research to inform teaching and contribute to the organizational research culture is, for some, a more productive activity than trying to become a (reluctant) research producer. This is clearly a matter for organizational determination.

This kind of research utilization is not confined to the educational setting. For any nurse, the process of thinking, reading and writing about research throws up interesting ideas, suggestions and new insights which, whilst not officially classed as 'findings' can be extremely valuable, perhaps providing the inspiration to test a new idea in practice or investigate a new topic. This personal interaction with research outputs can be seen as every nurse's opportunity.

We hope that, in this section, we have illustrated the need to analyse the complexity of what is meant by research utilization. Issues of who interprets the available findings, who synthesizes them with other sources of information and what skills are required to do this remain central and largely unresolved.

Research evaluator

CFRE defines the evaluator as 'One who has the skills to make and communicate judgements about the quality of the research and the strength of the evidence that arises from it'. This process is not the same as utilization of research although closely linked to it, often as a necessary preliminary step before the research output can be used to inform decisions.

Some authors are of the opinion that all nurses should be in a position to appraise the evidence in the available research literature. Docherty (2001) considers it the responsibility of each health care team member to critique the evidence before synthesizing it with other information. The demands of this mode of engagement with research are seen, by some, as modest: 'There is no great mystery about the ability to read research critically. Whilst it does require some knowledge, it is above all else a skill' (Freshwater, 2003). Statements like these fail to reveal the scope and range of the activities to which they refer. In theory, all professionals are required to engage with published research for educational and professional development purposes and be able to produce narrative literature reviews. Perhaps this is what is meant by the much used phrase 'critical reading' and can be seen as the baseline level for this mode of engagement. But the process of appraising the design, methods of data generation, analysis and interpretation relating to research in any particular field and then making judgements with any sort of practical implications requires greater expertise in both the methods and the substantive area. Although both could be said to engage with research in the evaluative mode, there is considerable difference between the level of engagement and the skills required in an interested reader and a person who reviews for professional purposes.

There is a further distinction which is sometimes overlooked. Other than the general critical reader, most research evaluators carry out the activity for a specific reason and with a particular product in mind. For example, a nurse working in an organizational development role may have the very specific task of assessing the evidence that has arisen from a set of previously conducted practice evaluations, to find out what can be learnt from the experience of others. Such a task demands a particular set of skills (Lyne *et al.*, 2002). The product of this activity will be influential in the local setting. At another level, the decisions reached by the nurse who acts as reviewer for a major journal will not have a direct influence on patient care in a locality, but may be very influential in the longer term. The work of journal reviewers affects what is published and therefore the content and quality of what is available to the utilizer community. It follows that such reviewers require appraisal and communication skills of an advanced, specialist nature. It could therefore be argued that some nursing roles demand particular sets of evaluative skills which may need to be accompanied by associated skills (such as communication and/or change management) in order to achieve a specified purpose. In other words, a profile of the required skills can be constructed.

In recognition of a general shortage of evaluative skills various types of critical appraisal methods and systems of training have been developed. These undoubtedly fulfil a very useful function in promoting a questioning approach, introducing appraisal methods and increasing practitioners' confidence and willingness to progress. But they tend to be provided in a 'one size fits all' model which fails to consider the requirements of the individual's role. The value of such systems is limited by the pre existing skills and work situation of the participants. For example, texts on appraisal methods frequently pose questions such as 'Are the nature of the population, the size of the sample and the definition of the variables given?' (Couchman and Dawson, 1995). The answer may be 'Yes, they are given, but I have no idea if they are OK'.

FoNS has been very active in efforts to get research into practice, organizing appraisal skills workshops throughout the UK. After assessing the impact of one series of workshops, FoNS found that over half the nurses lost their skills over time (The Foundation of Nursing Studies, 2001). A consultation exercise revealed that, in the opinion of the participants, the skills necessary to get research into practice were: people skills, evaluation skills, dissemination and leadership/management with the last being considered the most important. As a result of this study FoNS concluded that whilst critical appraisal skill was an important component of getting evidence into practice, other types of training are as, if not more, important.

As in the case of research utilization, these findings place a particular mode of research engagement in context as part of a network of skills. Moreover, they emphasize the need for clarity in terms of the level and purpose of research evaluation required for any role and the necessary educational preparation.

Research producer

The evaluators and users of research would be out of a job if it were not for those who conduct primary or secondary research and produce the varied outputs. Given the complexity of the first two modes of engagement which we have discussed, it comes as something of a relief to encounter a situation where the continuum of engagement is easier to describe, even if the skills required to undertake the various levels are not. However, when we start to look beneath the surface, we once again find areas requiring clarification, of which perhaps the most important is defining the baseline.

The research producer can be described as 'one who conducts primary or secondary research'. There have been strenuous efforts in nursing to demystify the conduct of research, because of its perceived inaccessibility to practitioners. This is laudable, but can be overdone, producing the impression that there's really nothing to it: 'research is really quite a friendly, everyday activity' (Couchman and Dawson, 1995). One view of research as part of nursing practice is that it is a skill, like others, which starts from a baseline and is developed over time, working from the foundation of a 'basic understanding of the research process' (Parahoo, 1997).

It is certainly true that descriptions of the 'research process' contain some very useful principles that provide a structure for all systematic methods of enquiry. They have intuitive attraction for nurses because of their similarities to the processes used in patient assessment, care planning and audit. But an understanding of this process is no more than a familiarity with a set of steps which describe in very broad (and oversimplified) terms some stages through which the conduct of research passes. It does not, in our view, convey any understanding of the reality of research, its demands and its rewards. We know of no other discipline that would regard an understanding of these processes as a baseline for research conduct. There is, therefore, a danger of assuming that, just as the new graduate nurse is ready to practice clinically, she/he is also equipped to carry out useful research. Unfortunately the analogy does not entirely fit, because a basic understanding of the research process is unlikely to be sufficient to enable the novice to do anything useful, except as an educational exercise. The development of skills which produce useful outputs in terms of research does not, under our current system of education, move at the same pace as the development of professional skills. The two are out of phase.

This is not to say that research carried out by relative beginners is never of practical use. There are and have been notable exceptions and the educational value may be considerable. But where research is identified as a component of a nursing role and is undertaken for a defined purpose, then quality is clearly an issue of paramount importance and it follows that appropriate skills are necessary.

The graduate or diplomate nurse leaving the educational system is in a position to produce a first synthesizing literature review, with supervision. With support, she/he can become involved in empirical work, either under supervision for educational purposes or acting in a technical capacity in an on going study, thus gaining sufficient experience to act as an independent data collector in a managed project. During this time the 'novice' research producer is acquiring a range of skills and techniques which contribute to the specialist methodological and substantive knowledge which is required of the independent investigator. Along with this, skills in writing, presentation and negotiation increase and knowledge of research politics and funding acquisition are enhanced. Ideally, this process of development should take place as part of a postgraduate programme. Finally, the experienced producer is recognized as an expert in a particular field with responsibility for securing research funding, designing projects, co-ordinating teams and all the additional functions of the career research leader. At this level, the research producer requires a range of skills in addition to research expertise. As we have seen in Chapter 2, in most disciplines attaining this level is a lengthy process, but in nursing the expectation is that it can be accelerated, from the artificially elevated baseline. It is true to say that nurses bring to this developmental process many additional skills and attributes, by virtue of their professional qualification and experience, and these certainly contribute to the desired profile and allow more rapid progress to be made in some aspects of research production. But they do not fill the gap between basic understanding and true expertise in research production. This is a nettle that, in our opinion, really needs to be grasped by the profession.

Research implementer

This mode of engagement spans individuals who implement research findings in their own practice through to those who implement research-based decisions in the development of policies and protocols at national level. In between, and of crucial importance, are those who implement research findings as they institute and manage change at department and organizational level.

The evaluation of research outputs and their subsequent use in decision making are processes that may appear to blend seamlessly with the implementation of research findings to inform policy and practice. However, we would argue that there are important differences. Whilst evaluation and utilization require capability in the interpretation and synthesis of evidence sources, implementation demands other skills, which come into play once the evaluators have appraised the evidence and the utilizers (who may of course, be the same people) have reached their decisions. For example, Studdart and Ramsden (2005) report their experience of introducing paediatric asthma clinical practice guidelines (CPG) into the Emergency Department (ED) of an Australian general hospital and conclude that:

> The introduction and implementation of CPG is not straightforward in any clinical setting. Combine this with a busy ED; introducing CPG into a non specialist ED; nursing shortages and junior medical staff who rotate regularly, then issues with implementation of CPG are confounded
>
> (Studdart and Ramsden, 2005, p. 3)

The skills involved here are those of leadership and change management, which are involved to an enhanced degree as the level of engagement with this aspect of research is raised from individual practice to the development and introduction of national policies and protocols. It could be argued that, for this purpose, these skills are much more important than expertise in research conduct and appraisal, as long as these capabilities are present within the system.

FoNS (2001) see the specialist or consultant nurse role as change agent and 'the bridge between the worlds of research and practice', indicating that implementation is yet another function of this role. Yet little attention has as yet been paid to this important mode of engagement, with most effort being directed towards the development of skills in the evaluation and conduct of research. As we will show in the following sections, the same is also true for the other identified modes of research engagement (teacher, supervisor, manager, influencer and leader). The skills needed for their performance remain under investigated.

Research teacher

The role of teacher is defined by CFRE as 'One who has expertise in certain types of research or aspects of the activity and transfers this to others'. In many academic disciplines, this transfer of expertise occurs through research based teaching in which the development of a subject is described through accounts of the research that has led to the present state of knowledge. Ideally, this is undertaken by research active academics deeply immersed in the literature of a particular field and, as the student progresses through their educational programme, they encounter teachers with greater and more specialised expertise. This teaching is coupled with formal instruction in the philosophy and ethics of research in that subject area and, where appropriate, with practical sessions on the techniques of subject specific inquiry. Thus the various aspects of the research activity and its products are integrated with the teaching of the subject matter so that the student becomes immersed in a research culture and familiarity with the concepts and principles of research is caught rather than taught.

As we have seen in Chapter 4, the range of subject matter covered by nurse researchers is very wide and therefore the above model is difficult to apply. There is also the continuing debate concerning what constitutes the discipline of nursing and therefore what can legitimately be identified as nursing research. These two issues produce some unique dilemmas for the profession, raising questions about how to teach the research component of professional practice and the skills required of those who engage with research in a teaching role. Further, since, as we are endeavouring to show in this book, the varied modes of research engagement within nursing are not yet clearly defined, the purpose of teaching the research component also remains unclear. Is the product of the activity to be the research user, producer, implementer, evaluator or all of these rolled into one? We suggest that there is a need for further consideration of these issues and a clearer specification of what is achievable by teachers of research at different levels and what expertise and experience they require to perform at these levels.

There is no disagreement that teachers of any element in the nursing curriculum require appropriate pedagogical expertise and this is assured through the quality systems in their institutions. As far as we are aware, there have been no investigations of the *relative* efficacy of various teaching and learning strategies in preparing learners to engage with research, although there have been evaluations of specific programmes (for example, Mulhall *et al.*, 2000) and this in our view, is an important gap in the literature. Veeramah (2004), having reviewed the literature in this area, concludes that there is 'very limited evidence on the effectiveness of research education provided through health related undergraduate programmes in the United Kingdom'.

The study reported by Veeramah was designed to evaluate an educational process in terms of the resultant self-reported attitudes to research, appraisal skills and use of research findings in practice, thus clearly placing the production of the combined research user and evaluator as the indicator of success. This is widely seen as the desirable outcome of undergraduate programmes, enabling the graduates to practise evidence-based health care (Hicks and Hennessy, 1994). If this is the case, two questions arise. First do the programmes fully achieve this purpose and second, how are nurses to be prepared for the other modes of engagement with research which constitute the network of skills on which success depends?

Veeramah's findings closely mirror those of earlier studies, in that whilst over 90 per cent of the respondents reported themselves as better prepared to appraise and use research findings on graduation, significant barriers to doing so were reported. These included lack of time (73 per cent), inability to understand statistical analyses (37 per cent) and lack of appraisal skills by colleagues (30 per cent). The first of these is identified by the author as an organizational issue which is unlikely to be resolved in the near future, and therefore makes it necessary for nurses to find the time for reading outside working hours. The second two are seen as deficits to be addressed by nurse educators, implying that it will be possible to bring everyone up to the desired level of expertise in both these areas. We have already stated our view that this is unattainable and the need for organizations to determine how they will ensure the presence and availability of appropriate expertise. We further suggest that research teachers have a much wider role to play in developing learners for the full range of roles within the network.

This brings us to the question of expertise. Apart from pedagogical skills, what preparation and experience is required to produce effective research teachers? What are the levels of performance within this domain? Can expertise in the subject matter be gained from theoretical study or is practical experience essential? Some clarity around these issues is really important because, as in all subject areas, the learner's attitude to the subject is likely to be influenced by the quality of the teaching and the mind set of the teacher.

In the diverse research arena of nursing the stance of the teacher has even more potential to influence the nature of the individual's research engagement. A strong preference for a particular philosophical position or approach to data generation can be communicated to students and set them off in a particular direction. This may be beneficial, leading to the development of specialised skills but on the other hand it may limit the choices available to the learner later on. Inspiring teaching can open new avenues and foster a latent interest in research but on the other hand sterile teaching can stamp out the early shoots of enthusiasm. Poorly informed teaching can give the learner a limited perspective on the subject and lead to a partial view of the nature, potential and demands of the research enterprise.

Ashworth *et al.* (2001) propose that various discourses exist within the nurse education community. In their investigation of what constitutes master's level performance they carried out in-depth interviews with 18 nurse lecturers teaching at this level throughout the UK. They interpreted the data to show the implicit discourses underlying the way that respondents discussed the attributes of master's graduates. One of these related to research orientation, revealing a 'tension between academic orientation and practical utility' and emphasizing the value of an appreciation of research findings as a route to good practice, but little more. The authors note the conspicuous absence of one possible discourse around research, i.e. the 'discourse of academic or intellectual achievement and personal growth as a valuable outcome of higher education in itself' (Ashworth *et al.*, 2001, p. 627). They conclude that the discourse of nurse lecturers mirrors current professional thinking and is likely to affect the profession in the future (hence their title 'Whither nursing').

In all these ways, the potential for research teachers to influence the research field in nursing can be seen and the fundamental importance of high quality, well informed teaching is made evident. However, because of the diversity of nursing research, provision of high quality research education is a more challenging task than it is in some other disciplines, where the field of subject matter has clearer boundaries and where the contribution of past research to the current state of the art has a longer and more visible history.

This challenge is illustrated by a recent debate on the contribution of quantative and qualitative methods to nursing research, which in itself provides an excellent source of teaching material for the more advanced student. Although this debate has been in progress for many years, an editorial by Watson (2003) rekindled the flames in a very interesting way. He argued for the primacy of scientific methods, meaning methods that involve replicable measurement and are thus objective, excluding any element of subjectivity from the processes of measurement and analysis and permitting subsequent replication, leading to confirmation or refutation. He then went on to dissect the claims of research which did not fulfil these criteria to any credibility or value. This, of course, produced a robust response from qualitative researchers. Draper and Draper (2003) take issue with Watson's assertions about the nature of science and subjectivity, arguing that all research methodologies should be valued for their potential to contribute to the advancement of knowledge when appropriately applied. Payne *et al.* (2003) adopt a view arising from the sociology of knowledge, that science is but one way of conceptualising the world and that all research is value laden, so that objectivity in science is a myth. They then effectively challenge his contention that qualitative studies are of little value by citing several seminal studies which have led to major changes in practice.

This debate contains excellent examples of logical argument and good humoured riposte, which enrich our research culture. We could do with more debate of this calibre. It also includes some unsupported contentions and, above all, evidence of a mutual lack of understanding of the opponent's position. Watson's insight into the nature of qualitative enquiry appears to be limited. It is, in many ways, a natural response of the scientist to the claims for scientific status which have been made by some qualitative nurse researchers. His opponents, on the other hand, display only a partial understanding of the nature of scientific enquiry and the consideration given by science to the acknowledged role of subjectivity in all fields of human activity. Reading the debate one receives the impression that the participants are 'divided by a common language', i.e. that they are using the same words but attaching different meanings to them.

This is only one of the current debates in nursing research, emphasizing the challenge for those who act in the teaching role. Is it possible for individuals to have a sufficient grasp, across all the diversity of this subject, to provide learners with opportunities to engage with these debates in a fully informed and therefore constructive manner? If not, does the limitation of our understanding as individual teachers help to propagate the sterility of some of these debates and slow our progress as a research-based profession? The logical conclusion of this line of thought would be the need for people who teach a research specialism within nursing, rather than nursing research as a subject.

Research supervisor

Many teachers also act as supervisors, but this mode of engagement with research requires an additional set of skills and, in nursing, has some distinctive characteristics which justify its separate consideration.

In the present context, the research supervisor is a person who acts in a supervisory capacity to less experienced research producers. The supervised work ranges from diploma level literature reviews, through undergraduate empirical projects to MPhil/PhD studies and finally to major research programmes carried out by career researchers. As in other fields of research, until comparatively recently there was an assumption that the possession of an academic qualification automatically brought with it the skills necessary for supervision at the level of that qualification. Recently the need to ensure quality and good governance in research degree programmes has been emphasized (HEFCE, 2003). More attention is now being given to the personal and intellectual attributes required and training schemes for supervisors have been put in place in most, if not all HEIs. The qualifications and experience required at every level are nowadays prescribed by academic institutions and bodies which fund research, so in this respect, academic supervision in nursing faces the same issues and challenges as supervision in any other discipline. However, because of the climate in which professional nursing takes place, there are some particular issues which affect the supervisory role. Very little literature exists in this field. Part II of this book contains some examples which illustrate these issues and the following section, based largely on the authors' own experiences, will attempt to bring them to the fore.

Within academic structures and professional research, the main explicit responsibility of the supervisor is to ensure that the supervisees' work achieves the criteria set for the course, programme of study or research programme. Throughout the continuum of engagement in this mode, and increasingly so at the higher levels, is implicit responsibility for supervisees', professional development and career progression, often leading to the establishment of research 'families' in which links with the supervisor are maintained throughout the career and continue into subsequent generations of researchers.

This is a relatively rare situation in nursing because of our limited supervisory capacity, prevailing discourses in nurse education and the nature of the pool of potential supervisees.

Thompson and Watson (2001) present a rather gloomy picture of research supervision in the UK, arguing that, after a promising start in the 1960s, academic nursing has suffered as a result of the expansion of higher education, shortened curricula and the managerial agenda, which emphasize the competencies in the curriculum at the expense of its more scholarly elements, such as research.

> Unfortunately, although the importance of research as an activity is increasingly being recognized, many nurses receive inadequate training, often compounded by poor supervision and mentorship.
>
> (Thompson and Watson, 2001, p. 2)

They do not cite data concerning the prevalence of observed or reported inadequate supervision, although there is certainly a wealth of anecdotal evidence of its occurrence. The sheer numbers of diploma, undergraduate and post registration students undertaking literature reviews and other projects places a severe burden on the supervisory capacity at these levels. Similarly, the increase in numbers of nurses undertaking higher degrees by research, and new postgraduate programmes with major research components have increased the demands for supervision at these more advanced levels (see Chapter 1).

A similar volume increase has occurred in many disciplines and, in itself is not the main source of the challenge faced by research supervisors in nursing. It is overlaid by the scarcity of people qualified to act in this capacity and the fact that the great majority of supervisees (apart from those in initial nurse education) are mature adults, often with considerable experience in and attachment to a particular area of nursing practice, education or management. This influences their preferred mode of learning; their selection of research topic; the processes of data generation; their interaction with colleagues and so on, in fact all of the elements of research in reality which are covered in Part 2 of this book. Several of the case studies presented there illustrate issues which need careful consideration by supervisors.

The earlier educational experience of the supervisees forms the basis for their initial approach to academic supervision. Although current programmes of nurse education are increasingly based on the principles of adult learning (O'Shea, 2003), in the past much of nurse education employed didactic, teacher centred methods (Nolan and Nolan, 1997). This, together with the realities of nursing practice, can lead to a preference for highly structured approaches to learning. Thompson and Sheckley (1997) present evidence from an American study to show that the mature students with nursing experience in their sample did indeed have this preference and in Chapter 9 of this book, Franklin describes her discomfort in moving from a highly structured clinical environment into the much more self-directed research setting.

The research supervisor, therefore, has to be prepared to deal with less experienced research producers whose expectations about the degree of structure and their own degree of autonomy as researchers vary considerably. There is no 'one size fits all' strategy and while it is natural for a supervisor who has experienced successful and enjoyable supervision to reproduce it, there is no guarantee that this will suit everyone. It is therefore very helpful to spend time exploring learning preferences, expectations and responsibilities at the very beginning of the supervisory period.

A particularly difficult transition for some nurse supervisees is that from being an expert in a particular field to being a complete novice as a researcher, especially if there are unrevealed gaps in the underlying knowledge base or unacknowledged deficits in skills which might be assumed to be present in a person operating at their professional level. Sometimes, these are the result of inadequate teaching at an earlier stage which has created a misunderstanding or block to learning which has never been resolved. (In our experience, strong men and women have been known to shed tears when confronted with relatively simple mathematical problems, others have expressed anger when being forced to apply logical reasoning and yet others have disappeared without trace when the supervisor has insisted on the production of some lucid writing. In deference to our own research supervisees we would point out that unresolved problems are always set against the wealth of experience and expertise which they bring to the research endeavour.) The supervisor sometimes has the difficult task of exposing these deficits, and helping the supervisee to acknowledge and seek to resolve them before their work can make real progress. This calls for assessment skills and experience of remedial methods at all levels in the supervisory mode of engagement.

In many cases, the selection of the project is determined by the supervisee and takes place within the context of that person's individual situation. In Chapter 6 below, Edmunds and Evans illustrate the dilemmas for aspiring nurse researchers when selecting topics which will satisfy a wide range of academic and professional concerns, a pressure which is much more strongly experienced in nursing than in many other disciplines. Guiding the student through this process and ensuring that the chosen topic has sufficient academic potential makes considerable demands on the time and skill of the supervisor, who needs to be able to appreciate the context and work with the student to realize the potential of their emergent ideas. Few nursing roles demand the use of a crystal ball, but perhaps this one is an exception, since the skilled supervisor is required to look into the future and foresee the likely direction of the proposed work, the evolution of the field of study and the possible risks to a successful outcome. The supervisor therefore needs to be very familiar with the work of others in the field, both past and present. As the level of supervision rises, the importance of this increases.

The attributes of the successful supervisor are often defined in terms of subject expertise, experience as a supervisee, procedural knowledge and a track record of successful project completions. Precisely what skills are used in successful day-to-day supervision is rarely defined and the elements of supervisory activity discussed above are rarely acknowledged and even more rarely costed. It is demanding and inevitably raises the question of how much time can and should be devoted to supervisory activity at any level. If nursing research is to make faster progress, should we adopt the model in which the ideal research students and project staff are self starting, flexible people with first class degrees, research training, boundless energy and uncomplicated lives? This might be an efficient solution. Or should we give more recognition to the pool of talent that undoubtedly exists in today's nursing workforce but which perhaps requires more supervisory input if that talent is to achieve its potential? This is a dilemma for both the individual supervisor and for those responsible for the strategic management of research in nursing.

Research manager

The managerial mode of engagement encompasses a spectrum of activity ranging from self-management by the research producer at any level through to management of international programmes and the commissioning of research at the highest levels. It encompasses both managing research and managing researchers; a subtle but important distinction as we will see later.

The baseline level for managing research is that of self-management by the person undertaking research. Apart from research competence, this requires skills in time management, goal setting, and project planning (Morrison and Burnard, 1990). For those nurses who engage with research as part of a wider professional role, it also calls for the ability to recognize and deal with role conflict, as several of our Part II case studies demonstrate.

These skills, if acquired at an early stage, are carried forward to the management of small and then larger research teams. Skills which need to be added to the repertoire are similar to those required in managing any team, perhaps including the multidisciplinary elements described by Sue Bale in her case study (Chapter 12). However, the management of researchers as team members presents some particular challenges that will be discussed at the end of this section.

Although research competence and experience are valuable for the team manager, their relative importance varies according to the nature of the project on which the team is working, especially in relation to its design and the volume and type of data produced. In the case of a project with a fully worked out protocol, such as a clinical trial, the main tasks for the manager of a single arm or a multi-centre study are organizational, e.g. recruiting and training data collectors; ensuring adherence to protocol and the principles of research governance; co-ordinating various team functions; recruitment and protection of subjects and so on. In contrast, the manager of a cross-site ethnographic study is faced with a much less predictable situation and, whilst still needing organizational and data management skills, is more likely to be called upon to engage with the evolution of the project over time and thus becomes involved in on going theoretical and methodological discussions.

Dealing with relationships within the project steering group and their interface with research staff is often an important role for the research manager and again, this varies according to the type of project and the composition of that group. So ideally the research manager should be able to reach an understanding of the priorities and agenda of the steering group as well as the constraints under which the researchers operate, the conditions necessary to maintain their motivation and morale and the strategies which can be used to support their career progression. In one sense, every project stands alone in that it involves a unique combination of agencies and individuals, with all their collaborating and sometimes competing interests and approaches to research. It is rare to find a job description for project manager which recognizes these elements of the particular piece of work, but given the pivotal role of manager we suggest that it would be advantageous to give more consideration to these specifications and the preparation of nurses for engagement with research in this way. (The role of trial co-ordinator is an exception to this statement, as the level of preparation and other requirements are usually well defined.)

From managing individual projects a natural progression is into an organizational role, either managing the research activity of a department; managing an element of research across the organization (for example research governance or research funding) or having responsibility for a commissioning function. These roles require the managerial and inter-personal skills described above with the addition of expertise in the necessary legal or policy frameworks, wider networks and greater intelligence concerning local, national and international policies and priorities. Political awareness and strategic planning skills assume increasing importance as the level of engagement rises.

The complexity of the context in which these roles are performed increases as the setting moves from local to national and beyond. Meerabeau (1996) provides an interesting perspective on the managerial role at this level in her account of her work as liaison officer in the UK government Department of Health where she had responsibility (with colleagues) for managing a national programme of health policy research. This involved the translation of governmental priorities into researchable questions and commissioning research teams to carry out projects which together would build the bigger picture needed to inform health policy. She points out the complexity of reconciling the requirements of several 'customers' (i.e. the three government departments that were working together in that policy area). Her role was to act as a bridge between the worlds of the policy makers and the health researchers, ensuring that the outputs from commissioned work would be academically rigorous. She quotes Kogan and Henkel (1983) to describe the attributes needed at this level. These included wide familiarity with the research field and its principal researchers; understanding of the world of health professionals who might be involved in any proposed research and knowledge of the workings of government departments. This demonstrates the breadth of intelligence required for successful operation at this level of research management. Expertise in a particular field of research production is not mentioned, rather this bridging role required sufficient familiarity with the overall research climate to know when to call in expert opinion.

Accounts such as this suggest a further discourse which we have not yet described and which is of particular relevance to the manager who has responsibility for the work of researchers; the discourse of the research community. We believe that managing research producers (as a distinct element of managing research activity) calls for some particular insights and this is important also for managers of nurses whose complex roles include any type of research engagement.

Managers in higher education sometimes liken their task to herding cats, implying that what they are trying to do is to gain some control over the activities of the ungovernable, particularly the researchers. Meerabeau (1996) draws attention to similar views held by some policy makers that researchers need to be controlled and their work focused to make it of use. These views imply a perceived reluctance on the part of researchers to direct their work towards desired outcomes. On the other hand, a former chief scientist at the Department of Health sees that researchers do not share the priority of policy makers for results with relatively short term utility.

> The views and needs of researchers are almost the exact converse. They do not want to be 'penny in the slot' responders: they wish to participate in the policy debate, and they want to develop long term plans and have time to speculate and innovate.
>
> (O'Grady, 1990, p. 2)

Meerabeau (1996) presents further views that researchers may not wish to become involved in the application of their work to inform policy, preferring to retain a stance which retains the purity of the work for its own sake. Lisa Franklin, in Chapter 9 of this book describes the differences she found between the thought processes of nurse clinicians and researchers. These and other sources point to a researcher mindset that is reflective, creative and wary of boundaries.

The impact of a highly managed approach to research is shown by the emergent responses to the RAE in UK academic institutions. Whilst, as we have shown in an earlier chapter, there have been some positive benefits for many disciplines, including nursing, such as the development of programmatic research, there have been casualties. Some researchers have found their work no longer valued because it did not fit the departmental profile and some have felt themselves subject to threats and bullying as their managers attempted to change the overall direction of their work (Lipsett, 2005).

The question for the research manager is how to ensure that research producers are able to conduct high quality work and, at the same time, meet the requirements of the organization or the customers. Clearly, the more managers understand the discourse of the research community, the more likely they are to succeed in this difficult balancing act. In addition, appreciating the variety of modes of engagement would assist managers to identify those who are best employed in each mode. Managing implementation, for example, presents a different challenge from managing the producers. A frequently cited barrier to research utilization is the lack of understanding by managers of the nature of research. Perhaps we have shown that one reason for the continual resurgence of this finding is a failure to analyse the components of research activity, to understand the skills and attributes needed by those who perform them and to use this information at all levels of the management of nursing roles which contain them.

Research influencer

The preceding discussion will, we hope, have illuminated the potential for nurses who engage with research in the various modes described to influence the success or failure of research activity within the profession. However, in the CFRE taxonomy, the mode of influencer has been identified in a particular way as 'one who contributes to the focus of research activity'. This implies that any nurse who takes part in discussions about research priorities or consultations around local research strategies is engaging with research in this mode. In that sense, all nurses can be research influencers, whether or not they engage in other ways. By identifying topics in need of study or questions in need of answers every nurse can influence the decisions which determine what research is prioritized, resourced and subsequently carried out.

However in order to do this, the influencer has to articulate the question or the precise nature of the topic in a way that the decision maker can understand. This sometimes proves to be challenging, resulting in research strategies which are so broad that they are not easily translated into action. We have often observed this to be the case in practice, but the reasons for this situation are unclear. We suggest that skills in the analysis and description of research topics or questions require more attention in the nursing curriculum, so that they become part of every nurse's skill set. In terms of the ability to influence the nature of nursing research, the widespread distribution of these skills could be more effective than attempts to spread producer and evaluator skills throughout the profession.

Being a research influencer, then, is potentially every nurse's business. For those who act as research producers, decisions of this nature are taken when beginning researchers make decisions about the direction of their own work, often with the guidance of supervisors as described above. Although it is not always obvious at the time, these decisions can be very influential in determining the shape of a future career through their effect on the initial experience of the researcher and their subsequent commitment to a particular approach or line of enquiry. As the career progresses, the researcher is likely to be involved in similar decisions concerning the research focus of teams and organizations, perhaps leading to the identification of priorities for investigation in their particular area of work. At the highest level for this mode of engagement comes participation in decision making and priority setting by national and international bodies.

Clearly the crucial skills here include the ability to access the necessary information and to make the best possible decision within the time available – in other words, as Linda Edmunds and Nicola Evans demonstrate in Chapter 6, to make and recognize a decision which is good enough for its purpose. Paradoxically, this can be more difficult at early stages, where the decision base appears to be infinite, than it is at the higher levels where the information needed is of a higher and more complex order but has clearer boundaries.

The commissioning of research is a further element of the influencer role, with nurses now becoming involved at earlier stages in their research careers, for example as members of research strategy committees within their organizations with responsibility for the disbursement of research monies to local projects. These bodies are, however, by definition competitive and the nurse representatives in a minority (often a minority of one) so that their ability to make a case that other committee members can appreciate is crucial. All members of the committee need the ability to determine which of the reviewed proposals are most likely to contribute to the designated purpose of the funds at the committee's disposal. This requires a high degree of professionalism and the absence of partisanship amongst the members, an ideal which, in our experience, is not always achieved. Mentorship and support for nurses who work in this way is very necessary, as it is for those who operate as members of commissioning bodies at the higher levels.

Scott and West (2001) present a cautiously optimistic picture of the increasingly legitimated involvement of nurses in the commissioning and priority setting processes. This has accompanied recent trends in research and health policy which have moved some way towards acknowledging new modes of knowledge production and the need for dedicated funding streams to support research other than clinical science, such as the Department of Health Service Delivery and Organization (SDO) programme (National Coordinating Centre for NHS Service Delivery and Organisation Research and Development, 1999). Their optimism is tempered by a number of caveats. First the concern that nurses will not wish to enter the broader arena and prefer to remain firmly located in purely nursing research. Second the lack of opportunities for the necessary training to support involvement at this level and finally the effect that reliance on the major funding bodies, such as the NHS, may have on the shape of nursing research.

The first two concerns reflect some of the dilemmas which have been already discussed in this book. The third demonstrates the need for nursing influence on the research agendas of the major funders. The skills required to exert this kind of influence are closely related to the final mode of research engagement which we will describe, that of research leadership.

Research leader

Some readers may be surprised to find that we have left this crucial mode of research engagement to the last. This has been done deliberately, since it was first necessary to set out the other modes and describe their complexity in order to make the requirements for leadership clear.

CFRE defines the research leader as 'One who has the vision for research, communicates it to others and develops a strategy for achieving it'. Now that we have described the network of modes of research engagement we hope that it is evident where these elements of leadership fit and how, as the level increases, the leader becomes engaged with more of the network components.

In the early stage, the research leader is responsible for the day-to-day running of a research project, maintaining its strategic direction by a clear vision of where the project is heading. Creating and sustaining that vision demands the ability to think widely and clearly. Progressing further the leader works at programme level, developing the strategic approach and leading by example as a producer of high quality research outputs. In addition to leadership skills such as delegation, the ability to motivate staff, and attention to detail, the programme leader engages with research as producer, utilizer, evaluator, manager and influencer, thus requiring the skills which we have defined already in addition to the clinical skills which may be required in some programmes. This is a very tall order, but is demanded of research leaders at middle levels in the leadership continuum, such as the nurse consultant or the university research group leader.

As the level increases, the research leader becomes more expert as a producer, moving to national and international levels of excellence and acquires responsibility for the leadership of larger research groupings, such as those of the unit, department and organization. The leader develops and sustains the vision for research within these groupings and assumes responsibility for strategic development to support that vision. In addition to the skill set already described, this leader requires the skills of the supervisor to nurture the research family and the political skills of the influencer in large measure. Above all, in order to maintain the vision, the leader should 'think big'. Thompson (2003) considers that the development of effective programmatic research in nursing is hampered by a lack of the leadership qualities of 'vision, strategy, focus, energy and confidence' as well as a shortage of ruthless ambition and political skills.

We are asking a great deal of our research leaders at both intermediate and higher levels. The importance of leadership training is increasingly recognized in service contexts and, perhaps more slowly, in HEIs. Generic leadership skills are promoted and valued, but the particular demands of research leadership are rarely addressed. Some rare individuals have already risen to these challenges and it is encouraging to see attempts to prepare outstanding people to engage with research in this way. But we consider that there is the need for much greater recognition of the difficulties which the present context of nursing creates for potential leaders and more active steps to deal with them.

Discussion

We hope to have demonstrated that it is possible (and useful) to unpick the web of research related activity to reveal the varied modes of engagement of which it is composed. It is important to emphasize that these modes and levels do not map directly onto professional roles; an individual may engage with research in one or more ways at any one time and over the course of the career the profile will change.

In several cases we have demonstrated the effect of underestimating the demands of the particular type of engagement. The roles of specialist and particularly consultant nurses appear to demand multiple modes of engagement, with a lack of clarity about the level of performance required. In a sense, these roles form the point of reference for all others. If we got this right the others would follow.

In the light of these ideas, we would argue that in nursing we have a sphere of 'proto research' in which the understanding of the nature of the activity, its demands and its deliverables is somewhat distorted. On the other hand, there is considerable expertise throughout the profession in functions such as change management, which are more essential for some modes on engagement. This results in an anomalous situation concerning the overall engagement with research of the profession, with some people being expected to do more than is necessary and others expected to perform functions for which they are unprepared.

References

Allen, D., Lyne, P., Watkins, D., Taylor, S., Proctor, S. and Gill, P. (2004) *The Cardiff Framework of Research Engagement*, Cardiff: University of Wales College of Medicine.

Ashworth, P.D., Gerrish, K. and McMannus, M. (2001) 'Whither nursing: discourses underlying master's level performance in nursing', *Journal of Advanced Nursing*, 34, 621–8.

Couchman, W. and Dawson, J. (1995) *Nursing and Healthcare Research: A Practical Guide*, London: Scutari.

Di Censo, A., Cullum, N. and Ciliska, D. (1998) Editorial: 'Implementing evidence based nursing: some misconceptions', *Evidence Based Nursing*, 1, 38–40.

Docherty, B. (2001) 'The nursing contribution to evidence based practice', *Nursing Progress*, 10; http://www.rlhleagueofnurses.org.uk/Education/Nursing_Progress/Issue10/NursingEBP/nursingebp.html

Draper, J. and Draper, P. (2003) 'Response to Watson's guest editorial', *Journal of Advanced Nursing*, 44, 546–7.

Fawcett, J. (2003) Guest editorial: 'On bed baths and conceptual models of nursing', *Journal of Advanced Nursing*, 44, 229–30.

Feynman, R.P. (2005) *Don't You Have Time to Think.* Edited and with additional commentary by Michelle Feynman, London: Allen Lane.

Freshwater, D. and Bishop, V. (2003) *Nursing Research: Appreciation. Critique and Utilisation*, Basingstoke: Palgrave.

Funk, S.G., Tornquist, E.M. and Champagne, M.T. (1995) 'Barriers and facilitators of research utilization: An integrative review', *Nursing Clinics of North America*, 3, 395–408.

Gething, L. and Leelarthaepin, B. (2000) 'Strategies for promoting research participation among nurses employed as academics in the university sector', *Nurse Education Today*, 20, 147–54.

HEFCE (2001) *Promoting Research in Nursing and the Allied Health Professions: Research Report 01/64*, London: Higher Education Funding Council England.

—— (2003) *Improving Standards in Postgraduate Research Degree Programmes*, Formal consultation: Department for Employment and Learning, Northern Ireland; HEFCE: Higher Education Funding Council for Wales; Scottish Higher Education Funding Council. London: Higher Education Funding Council England.

Hicks, C. and Hennessy, D. (1994) 'Quality in post-basic nurse education: the need for evidence based provision', *Journal of Nursing Management*, 7, 215–24.

Kirshbaum, M., Beaver, K. and Luker, K. (2004) 'Perspectives of breast care nurses on research dissemination and utilisation', *Clinical Effectiveness in Nursing*, 8, 47–58.

Kogan, M. and Henkel, M. (1983) *The Rothschild Experiment in a Government Department*, London: Heinemann.

Lipsett, A. (2005) 'Bullying rife in run up to RAE', *Times Higher Educational Supplement*, 21 October.

Lyne, P., Allen, D., Satherley, P. and Martinsen, C. (2002) 'Improving the evidence base for practice: a realistic method for appraising evaluations', *Journal of Clinical Effectiveness in Nursing*, 6, 81–8.

Marsh, G., Nolan, M. and Hopkins, S. (2001) 'Testing the revised barriers to research utilization scale for use in the UK', *Clinical Effectiveness in Nursing*, 5, 66–72.

Meerabeau, E. (1996) 'Managing policy research in nursing', *Journal of Advanced Nursing*, 24, 633–9.

Morrison, P. and Burnard, P. (1990) *Nursing Research in Action: Developing Basic Skills*, Basingstoke: Macmillan Press.

Mulhall, A., Le-May, A. and Alexander, C. (2000) 'Research based nursing practice – an evaluation of an educational programme', *Nurse Education Today*, 20, 435–43.

National Coordinating Centre for NHS Service Delivery and Organisation Research and Development (1999) *National Listening Exercise – Interim Report on the Findings*, London: NCCSDO London School of Hygiene and Tropical Medicine.

Nolan, J. and Nolan, M. (1997) 'Self-directed and student centred learning in nurse education 1', *British Journal of Nursing*, 6, 51–5.

O'Grady, J. (1990) 'Valediction', in *Department of Health Year Book on Research and Development 1990*. London: Department of Health.

O'Neill, E., Dluhy, N., Fortier, P. and Michel, H. (2004) 'Knowledge acquisition and validation: a model for support systems', *Journal of Advanced Nursing*, 47, 134–42.

O'Shea, E. (2003) 'Self-directed learning in nurse education: a review of the literature', *Journal of Advanced Nursing*, 43, 62–70.

Parahoo, K. (1997) *Nursing Research: Principles, Process and Issues*, Basingstoke: Macmillan Press.

Payne, S., Seymour, J. and Ingleton, C. (2003) 'Response to Watson's guest editorial', *Journal of Advanced Nursing*, 44, 547–8.

Rycroft-Malone, J., Seers, K., Titchen, A., Harvey, G., Kitson, A. and McCormack, B. (2004) 'What counts as evidence in evidence based practice?', *Journal of Advanced Nursing*, 47, 81–90.

Scott, C. and West, E. (2001) 'Nursing in the public sphere: health policy research in a changing world', *Journal of Advanced Nursing*, 33, 387–95.

Stinson, S. (2004) Personal Communication at University of Alberta Hospital.

Studdart, J. and Ramsden, C. (2005) 'Introduction of standardised emergency department asthma clinical guidelines into a general metropolitan hospital', *Accident and Emergency Nursing*, 13, 2–8.

The Foundation of Nursing Studies (2001) *Taking Action: Moving Towards Evidence Based Practice*, London: The Foundation of Nursing Studies.

Thompson, C. and Sheckley, B. (1997) 'Differences in classroom teaching preferences between traditional and adult BSN students', *Journal of Nursing Education*, 36, 163–70.

Thompson, D. (2003) Editorial: 'Thinking bigger about research', *Journal of Advanced Nursing*, 43, 1–2.

Thompson, D. and Watson, R. (2001) Editorial: 'Academic nursing – what is happening to it and where is it going?', *Journal of Advanced Nursing*, 36, 1–2.

Traynor, M. and Rafferty, A.M. (1998) *Nursing Research and the Higher Education Context: A Second Working Paper*, London: Centre for Policy in Nursing Research, London School of Hygiene and Tropical Medicine.

Veeramah, V. (2004) 'Utilisation of research findings by graduate nurses and midwives', *Journal of Advanced Nursing*, 47, 183–91.

WAG (2004) *Realising the Potential: Briefing Paper 6: Achieving the Potential Through Research and Development. A Framework for Realising the Potential Through Research and Development in Wales*, Cardiff: Welsh Assembly Government.

Watson, R. (2003) Editorial: 'Scientific methods are the only credible way forward for nursing research', *Journal of Advanced Nursing*, 43, 219–20.

Part II

The reality of nursing research

Tales from the field

Introduction

Having set out the context for nursing research and described the factors shaping the current situation, we now turn our attention to the real world of nursing research practice. Through a series of case studies we aim to show how nurse researchers have experienced the impact of these interacting factors on their work and to share some of the strategies developed to deal with them.

The case studies have been selected to illustrate the stages through which the conduct of research passes, from selection of topic to dissemination of findings, and the impact of the varied discourses described in Part I. Although there are several textbooks which describe these stages, it is unusual to have the opportunity to read such first-hand accounts written by those involved.

Biographical details of the authors can be found at the beginning of this book. Each case study is written in the first person, authors are referred to informally, by their first names and, although the chapters have been edited to ensure consistency throughout the book, the style of each account preserves that of the author as far as possible. This, we hope, makes Part II a vivid and varied collection of real experiences.

Chapter 6

Selecting a topic

Nicola Evans and Linda Edmunds

Introduction

We begin Part II at what seems to be a logical point: the selection of the topic for a research project or programme. In many cases, this first occurs when a new graduate begins the process of registering for a higher degree and is clearly a critical and influential step in the development of a research career. More experienced researchers face this kind of choice at several stages in their careers, when deciding whether to continue an existing line of research or switch to something else. Here the selection is informed by a greater knowledge of the research field and its context, together with personal and domestic considerations and attention to the consequence for career development. In nursing, most people who come to this point, as graduate students or otherwise, have experience of professional life and are embedded in its culture. So added to all the other factors influencing the decision are the varied discourses and values that have been described in Part I. The aim of this chapter is to illustrate this complexity by drawing on the experience of two novice researchers who were deciding upon a topic for their first major research studies. Research methods texts vary in the extent to which they give attention to this crucial phase (Parahoo, 1997; Silverman, 2000). However, we have found that the process involves some totally unforeseen aspects, as illustrated by the two case study examples below. These are presented as reflexive analyses of the process of selecting a researchable topic.

> **Case study 1: Establishing a research portfolio – Linda**
> The consultant nurse role has five components: expert practice, leadership, service development, teaching and research. On being appointed to my current post as Consultant Nurse, Cardiac Care, I felt prepared to take on many of its challenges, having clinical expertise and experience of service development, leadership and teaching. However, I was aware of a need to develop the research component. Throughout my career I had always believed that good practice is based upon research and evaluation, and had been engaged with research through disseminating findings and encouraging critical thinking, but had little experience of conducting research myself. When I took up the post I was seven months into a Public Health MSc. This was a three-year course, consisting of themed modules (including one on research methodology) with the third year focused on the dissertation. It was this which provided me with the opportunity to develop my first independent research project.

When I had been in post for approximately six months I took time to reflect on the development of my role and initially was concerned that the research element was weak. However, after further consideration I realized that, there had been a great deal of 'research mindedness' taking place in the form of observation, questioning, reading and above all thinking (Parahoo, 1997). I also found that undertaking my MSc helped me to focus my reading and explore the literature in more depth than I had in the past. It was the early literature exploration that raised many questions for me around coronary heart disease prevention and it was during the early part of my MSc that I started to formulate and think about initial ideas for my choice of topic. However, my thinking was being shaped by a range of other concerns, although at the time I was almost unaware that this was taking place.

From the time that I came into post, I was conscious that I needed to exert influence on both strategic and clinical developments as part of my role, which was focused around the recommendations of *Tackling Coronary Heart Disease in Wales* (National Assembly for Wales, 2001). This Welsh Assembly Government document sets out the framework to provide the 'gold standard' of expected care for cardiac patients. My inclination was for my research to be related to the expected outcomes within the framework, reflecting both aspects of my role; strategic development and clinical practice. However, the framework is very target driven, presenting outcomes in terms of numbers and timescales, and offering little advice on best practice. I became concerned because short-term projects were being developed within the organization to meet these targets, for example, clinics to reduce the risk of coronary heart disease, without any reference to the relevant evidence base. I considered that it was important to understand the factors contributing to the success of such interventions as well as to measure the achievement of targets. For several years I had been interested in the impact of patients' beliefs on the outcomes of care and in particular, their understanding of the nature of their condition and their preferences regarding the best person to provide ongoing care. I therefore made this my first choice of broad study area.

Nevertheless, feelings of doubt and uncertainty lingered. I felt there were expectations from my employers that I should focus on strategic issues and that they would not share my belief that patients' understanding was fundamental to these. To deal with this uncertainty, I decided that I needed criteria to confirm the suitability of my choice. I established objectives that I required the research findings to achieve. These were: to contribute to the overall reduction of coronary heart disease mortality and morbidity; to support the delivery of evidence-based models of risk factor reduction; to assist patients and the public to influence the delivery of health care and to provide insight into patients' understanding of their condition and its management. After considerable reflection and critical conversations with colleagues, I was confident that the chosen subject area did indeed have a strategic and clinical focus and fit the criteria that I had set. My conviction that the overall targets of reducing cardiac mortality and morbidity could only be achieved if attention is paid to the details of service delivery was strengthened.

A key learning point for me was the recognition of the many external influences which impacted on this initial choice of subject and resulted in the need to ensure that it satisfied several important requirements of my role, i.e. that it was 'fit for purpose'. Having recognized and acknowledged these influences, I was in a stronger position to control the development of my research question and to resist any pressure from external influences that did not make connections with my internal beliefs. Another learning point for me was that the process of topic selection requires considerable time, during which the relationship between internal and external influences can be worked through. It was only after taking the time to do this that I became confident that my chosen subject did indeed 'fit' with strategic developments and I was therefore better able to justify the choice to others.

Having fixed upon this broad area of interest, I needed to narrow the subject area down and identify a specific question. To do this I initially responded to my own 'gut instinct': I believed that nursing had an important role in delivering cardiac care and in particular in the delivery of secondary prevention (i.e. reducing risk factors for coronary heart disease through lifestyle changes and/or drug therapy). Despite the evidence that secondary prevention is effective at reducing mortality and morbidity of coronary heart disease (EUROASPIRE I and II Group; European Action on Secondary Prevention by Intervention to Reduce Events, 2001), my observations of clinical practice indicated that approaches are varied and that health professionals are not always effective in achieving the secondary prevention targets set within the national framework. The question I came back to was: Why are we not successful in reaching these secondary prevention targets? It was from here that I returned to the earlier reading in my career and the literature studied throughout my MSc and looked at secondary prevention in more detail.

There are many aspects to secondary prevention including the evidence base for treatment, delivery of intervention, social influences and concordance with treatments, but the area that took my interest was the potential impact of an individual's understanding of their illness and the effect this may have on their recovery. As my exploration of the topic continued I extended my search beyond the nursing literature into the social sciences, public health and medicine. In the health psychology literature I used key words such as 'illness perception' and 'lifestyle change' and discovered a paper by Petrie et al. (1996), which dealt with the impact of patients' beliefs on recovery and lifestyle, demonstrating that very simple changes to the way we share information and check our understanding can have a significant impact on recovery, which was clearly central to my area of interest. This influenced my final choice of topic for my MSc dissertation, to which I gave the title 'A study to identify patients' perception of their heart condition, support for lifestyle changes and the health professional best placed to manage their care'. After taking time to consider the many drivers influencing my choice and setting criteria for my selected topic I now felt comfortable that my topic had a strategic and clinical focus, gave proper prominence to patient involvement, and sought to challenge existing ineffective service provision.

Returning repeatedly to the literature helped to make sense of my ideas and instincts. It was an ongoing process that continually shaped my thoughts and refined my area of interest, becoming of fundamental importance to my final topic choice. Previously I viewed the literature review as a stand-alone component of the research process, and this is how it is sometimes presented, but this can be very limiting in the selection of a topic. Clinical experience, experiential knowledge and reviewing the literature I consider are all entwined together, one feeding off the other and producing more questions to be answered. I believe this connection of practice, knowledge and literature reviewing is what forms the foundation for future and present work.

It proved to be important to develop a wide review of literature including other disciplines, and covering a variety of research methods. This provided a greater depth of understanding in the research topic area. However, in the real world this cannot be an open-ended process and there is clearly a need to come to a final decision and commit to a chosen topic. I realized that, in my case, I was ready to commit when I was sure that the chosen subject did fit with the pre-defined criteria, i.e. that the findings would have the potential to influence the identified key issues. I recognized this when I felt confident and competent when justifying my choice of research topic to colleagues and critical friends. At this stage of the process I had shared my developing ideas with a range of interested people, former clinical colleagues (not those who would be affected by any proposals from the research), lecturers and senior nursing colleagues.

After completing the project I began to see that it could form the basis of ongoing research and practice change and that I would need to share my findings with affected colleagues – both clinicians and managers – to secure their cooperation. Clinicians within the field had been supportive throughout my project and were interested in my study and yet I found it difficult to present them with findings that suggested the need for change without having involved them at an earlier stage. I was concerned that they would view it as a criticism of current practice. When I did share my work with colleagues their initial response was that there was a lot of information for them to take on board all at once. I felt they would not accept the recommendations for practice until they understood the thinking behind the project and how it had taken place. When sharing my findings with managers a similar scenario took place where I had to ensure they understood how the study linked with strategic issues. It was only at this stage they understood the relevance of the findings. This made me realize the importance of engaging with stakeholders throughout the process. On reflection the development of a research group to 'bounce' ideas off would have been invaluable in refining the topic for study and through this engage stakeholders, managers and clinicians at an early stage so that the research would be considered as an integral part of care and not as a separate 'project'.

During the development of a research topic, the consultant nurse has to interact with a wide range of interested parties, all of whom will be affected by the choice. The way in which the developing topic is presented to these different groups may need to vary and there is a need to 'package' the topic demonstrating where it fits with strategic and local policy, professional agenda and the potential implications for practice. Therefore thought needs to be given as to how the findings will be acted upon and stakeholders proactively enrolled in the process to enable this to happen. This issue highlights the need for all nurse researchers to ensure that research proposals are discussed at an early stage with managers and clinicians through a clinical governance agenda. Many other disciplines when choosing a research study only have to consider if the research is 'doable', however in nursing there are many other influences. Nurses have to consider how the research is valued, the impact it may have on services, and the relationship with practice and other health professionals.

Case study 2: Shifting sands – Nicola

Having worked in two specialist fields of mental health nursing – forensic and child and adolescent mental health services (CAMHS) – I moved into a lecturing position after considerable soul searching about the consequences of moving away from direct patient care. Once I decided to take an academic position, I was determined to retain clinical credibility in the field, and maintain real links with practice. One option, which I pursued for a year, was to do a small amount of clinical work each week for a local NHS Trust. The other was the development of a research project addressing practice issues in my chosen speciality, a process which is ongoing at the time of writing.

Before starting on the journey of selecting a topic, I had anticipated that it would be a linear, logical progression. This may be the case for some people. However, I discovered that it is a cyclical process of certainty and uncertainty, knowing and not knowing, clarity of thought and confusion about the precise nature of the subject matter. The process of selecting a topic is subject to a number of factors that interact in an unpredictable fashion, factors that emerge from inside the researcher; ideas, aspirations, expectations, and ideas that originate from the environment; priorities, expectations of others, and funding opportunities.

While bedding in to my new post at the university I decided that, in terms of career pathway, I was in a prime position to develop my research skills further by registering for a PhD. I wanted to integrate the two strands of my previous clinical experience into a topic for a substantial research project. This, I reasoned, would define my career to this point as the product of a strategic professional developmental plan that showed vision, by bringing together significant pieces of previous work. I had previously completed a Criminology MSc and had undertaken a qualitative study addressing factors relating to prisoners' mental health. My more recent clinical practice had been with children with mental health problems. It therefore seemed logical to bring the two strands together by researching the health component of services for children who offend. I also believed this development of a research plan would give my PhD proposal evidence of sustained thought and credibility and thus increase the likelihood of its acceptance as a feasible higher degree study.

After I had been in post for nine months the opportunity for me to have a short research secondment arose. I planned to use this to develop further the idea for my PhD by conducting a literature review on the impact of a specialist health worker service on the mental health of young offenders, having reached agreement that this broad area was congruent with the school's strategic research focus. As I began to search the literature, I quickly realized this was indeed uncharted territory, with little published or unpublished research. Although this confirmed that the topic was ready for exploration and hence a potentially fruitful area in which to work, I found that my enthusiasm for it rapidly waned and I became concerned about whether I would be able to sustain an interest for the duration of a long haul research project or, indeed, for a programme of work emanating from the PhD. I began to realize that, if I was to move forward, I would have to take a step back, re-think my priorities and let go of this topic.

During this period I had conversations with clinical colleagues and colleagues currently engaged in research. Some questioned my choice on the grounds that it was a considerable departure from my clinical focus on mental health services for children and young people. Others queried whether it would sustain my interest into the future. I found myself involved in an intense internal debate around ownership, whether I should stand my ground about my original thinking, or whether I should be swayed through feedback from others. Reflecting on this part of my case study, I am reminded of one aspect of JoHari's window (Luft, 1969) – what others know but you do not. Others noticed in me the lack of connection between my intended research study and my original area of clinical interest before I did, but the transition to acquiring this knowledge was a difficult one. Other elements in this debate were the strength of my commitment to the chosen subject and the impact on others of any changes which might be made. The proposed study was about to become part of my life for the next five years. I needed this therefore to be complementary to other working roles in a constructive way as well as creating a springboard for future career development.

I carefully thought about the effect that any change of focus would have on my developing reputation. I had significant anxieties about becoming associated with the practice of incomplete projects, muddled thinking, lack of vision or focus and an inability to achieve clarity within the context of project planning as I had no history with the organization that could challenge such attributions. I also worried that I would damage the developing supportive relationships that I was building with colleagues within the Research Centre, who may have felt their time spent with me on my initial idea had been wasted. Despite all these concerns, I realized that I had to take the difficult decision to let go of my commitment to this topic and consider alternatives. This proved to be crucial in allowing me to move my thinking forward to achieve a satisfactory resolution about my topic choice.

I returned to a topic in which I had been previously interested and which had remained at the back of my mind. In my clinical post in CAMHS, I had become increasingly frustrated about the operation of the waiting list system. Appointments were allocated on the basis of referral letters which did not accurately describe the severity of the patients' problems. Therefore the waiting list did not reflect the priority of the patients' needs. The whole system needed a redesign and I decided to transfer my focus of interest to the problem of remedying the defects in this system.

In order to convert this interest into a researchable topic, I again discussed my ideas with trusted colleagues. Their feedback helped create the outline for a possible clinical project. I met the leader of a CAMHS team to explore whether we could develop the project idea and together considered ways that the waiting list could be tackled. At this stage, the triage idea emerged. Triage is a term used for quickly assessing and prioritizing the order in which people are seen in a service. Research supervision promoted the translation of this idea into a methodologically sound action research project which was subsequently developed into a successful application to a major funding organization committed to leading practice through research. Feedback during this process fine-tuned the project until a final product was achieved.

The final selection of the research topic and the choice of action research to address the waiting list issue satisfied a number of important conditions. It was congruent with my personal belief that practice is an essential component of my work; it allowed for the integration of teaching, research and clinical practice into a research proposal that met my personal objectives; it fitted with the academic department's research strategy in terms of themes and practice foci, and fitted with the political climate and the Welsh Assembly Government's research priority areas of mental health and children and young people (WAG, 2004).

The choice of topic proves to be a dance at the interface between personal choice and external driving forces. Negotiating access to a clinical area, collaborating with a clinical, management and academic supervisory team created layers of dialogue that challenged my original focus for the project. The debate at these junctures revolved around whether to stick rigidly to my own idea or to be persuaded by stakeholders to blend their ideas within my own. Clearly there were risks associated with both approaches. Too much rigidity may convey to the stakeholders my general lack of flexibility, and thus affect their preparedness to accommodate practice changes, or new ideas. Too much accommodation of others' ideas and my project would become too unwieldy to remain feasible.

Contributing to new knowledge about a topic area is a key requirement for doctorate level study. Finding that area of personal interest within political and professional parameters, whilst being mindful of developing an area of new knowledge, creates an internal dialogue between yearning to 'discover' a new model/method of work and the anxieties about length, breadth and size of project. Without experience of knowing how much time and resource a project takes and without informed supervision the topic selected may outstretch available resources and the student fail to complete. Supervision cannot start early enough. It helped in the formation and germination of the project idea as did exposure to critical friends who posed pivotal questions that demanded a degree of reading and reflection before answers could be provided. It also gave me permission and reassurance that taking time to 'think' was not only a legitimate activity, but an essential precursor to high quality research.

Discussion

Despite our very different experiences and situations, similar themes emerge from the two case studies which provide useful learning points.

Understanding the multiple factors influencing the process

As Part 1 of this book has shown, clinical nurses acting as research producers are subject to a number of influences and are caught in the middle of the academic and practitioner agenda in addition to the political and management agenda. Both case studies have identified how the researchers, at differing times, felt the impact of internal and external influences on their subject choice. In the first case study, Linda felt the external pressures of role expectation, employers and peer expectations. Nicola, in the second case study, experienced external pressures in the form of the need to maintain credibility in both clinical and academic fields and to establish a position within an organization. Internal influences for both researchers emerged as passion for the subject area, belief in the value of the topic to be studied as well as personal issues relating to time and support mechanisms. We found that acknowledging and naming all these influences or drivers, produced an understanding of their respective significance and enabled each of us to identify the most important criteria on which to base our choice of research topic. It became apparent that each of us had done this almost unconsciously. We generated some of these criteria and others emanated from the requirements of significant people or organizations. For example, when considering applying for funding, Nicola took into account the basis on which the funding application was likely to be judged and tailored her application to maximize chances of success.

In writing this chapter we produced a spider graph or map of these drivers from a series of brainstorming exercises. This visual representation helped us to understand how drivers were positioned in relation to one another, to understand their origin and strength of influence and thus to control their contribution to the final decision. On reflection, it is interesting to observe the differences between these maps in our two cases, suggesting that each research opportunity creates a different map. We noticed that these relationships were dynamic so as the relationship with one driver changed this had a consequential effect on other factors. Such a map can be linked to a career or personal plan to help predict how the choice of topic is going to affect future opportunities and prospects. This may provide the rationale for the choice of a topic which appears more problematic at present than others but has the potential to generate, for example, an exciting long-term prospect of change in services or a desired career move. It may also provide a useful aid to methodological transparency, enabling the researcher to be clear about how topic selection was decided. These processes can be difficult to retrieve from memory when writing a research report several years later.

Passion and excitement

One of the most critical drivers that emerged was that of passion or excitement for the subject. The idea of 'being excited' by the research area showed itself differently for each of us. Given the amount of work involved in developing an idea into a research proposal and then full project, there are significant advantages to having a sense of enjoyment when doing the work. The relationship between the project and researcher needs therefore to have a degree of 'excitement' to initiate the project but for the relationship to be sustained over time, the project needs to fit with core values. Delamont and Atkinson (2004) flag this point when underlining the need for the student to develop a researchable project and to see it as a necessary stepping-stone on the path to a research career, rather than the final word on a subject. What constitutes a do-able project will reflect the context in which the project is located for the individual concerned.

The evolution of ideas and knowing when to stop

The final researchable idea evolved over time for both case studies. The process of writing, reading, thinking, and re-writing produced a progressive definition of the research topic, increased confidence in its suitability and improved our ability to respond to critical questioning. Having the courage to expose developing ideas to critical friends proved to be essential. Amongst other things, this helped us both to improve our skills in articulating ideas succinctly and appropriately for diverse listeners. Sometimes it also exposed areas where things had been assumed or taken for granted and we had to think them through.

This evolutionary process takes time and we were interested to find that, in both cases, we recognized the need to create a balance between taking sufficient care to identify a feasible and productive topic and spending infinite amounts of time to get the 'perfect' one. We both knew when to stop, or, in other words, when the research idea was 'good enough'. On reflection we were able to identify that this stage was reached when we were aware of our confidence in the emerging project idea. This was reflected in our ability to envisage how the project would be carried out, our confidence in responding to critical review and challenges to the underlying thinking and our recognition that the final idea was congruent with original thinking and our core values.

Ensuring fitness for, and clarity of, purpose

Given all the influences affecting the choice of research topic, it may be difficult to discern the true purpose for which the work is being carried out. We both had to deal with a multiplicity of purposes. For example, Linda had commenced a new role, which included the expectation that she would undertake research. However, the role of consultant nurse focuses on the modernization and development of services at both a strategic level and the point of provision of clinical services. Therefore it was essential that the research reflected the organization's strategic direction as well as being designed to improve the delivery of care. At that time in her career she felt that if there was too strong an emphasis in either direction, strategic or service delivery, then credibility of the role could be jeopardized. The purpose of the research was therefore to satisfy both of these requirements, as well as providing her with necessary research experience.

In the second case study the purpose of the research was to cement the interaction between education, research and clinical practice. The topic of the research project therefore needed to emerge from the clinical domain. It also needed to offer the potential for the basis of a cumulative knowledge base making a significant contribution to academic debate in the field, as it was to be the focus for a PhD study. The purpose again was multi-faceted and driven by a combination of internal and external driving forces that required reconciliation to create a researchable topic that met the research purpose. Clearly, the purposes relate to the many influences or drivers that we have described above. We found that the map of the drivers was helpful in clarifying purpose and enabling us to keep sight of what were for us the true purposes guiding our choice of topic. The key question 'Just *why* am I doing this?' was one to which we were impelled to return frequently and we needed to revisit our reasoning periodically.

Engaging with stakeholders

Although this theme links with the previous three themes, it is worthy of discussion in its own right. To the novice researcher (and sometimes, it appears, to the more experienced as well) the value of identifying and engaging stakeholders is not obvious. We both gained an appreciation of its importance, but in rather different ways, Linda through reflection after completion of the study and Nicola through experience of very helpful stakeholder input during the planning stage. We have concluded that if the purpose of the research is to have a direct impact upon any system of practice, the inclusion of the relevant stakeholders at the initial stage of choosing the topic is essential, although it may result in a period of being sidetracked or even re-definition of the research idea.

Conclusion

In nursing, many interacting factors influence the selection of topic, more than in most other areas of work. The time and skills needed to navigate a course through this complex territory are often underestimated. These case studies suggest strategies which can be employed to make this complexity more manageable.

References

Delamont, S. and Atkinson, P. (2004) *Successful Research Careers: A Practical Guide*, Buckingham: Open University Press.

EUROASPIRE I and II Group; European Action on Secondary Prevention by Intervention to Reduce Events (2001) 'Clinical reality of coronary prevention guidelines: a comparison of EUROASPIRE I and II in nine countries', *The Lancet*, 357, 995–1001.

Luft, J. (1969) *Of Human Interaction – The JoHari Model*, Palo Alto, CA: Mayfield.

National Assembly for Wales (2001) *Tackling Coronary Heart Disease in Wales*, Cardiff: National Assembly for Wales.

Parahoo, K. (1997) *Nursing Research: Principles, Process and Issues*, Basingstoke: Macmillan Pres.

Petrie, K.J., Weinman, J., Sharpe, N. and Buckley, J. (1996) 'Role of patients' views of their illness in predicting return to work and functioning after myocardial infarction: a longitudinal study', *British Medical Journal*, 312, 1191–4.

Silverman, D. (2000) *Doing Qualitative Research: A Practical Handbook*, London: Sage Publications.

WAG (2004) *Realising the Potential: Briefing Paper 6: Achieving the Potential through Research and Development: A Framework for Realising the Potential through Research and Development in Wales*, Cardiff: Welsh Assembly Government.

Chapter 7

Negotiating a proposal through gate-keeping committees

Davina Allen and Ben Hannigan

Introduction

One of the many hurdles any researcher is required to overcome is the need to navigate a project proposal through a series of powerful gate-keeping committees. In the UK, the most significant of these are: grant awarding bodies, independent NHS research ethics committees, and NHS trust research governance committees. Whilst each has different functions, the challenges they present are very similar. In this chapter we examine these processes, drawing on our experiences of developing an application for research funding and securing research ethics approval for two studies which shared the same design. We conclude by analysing the lessons arising from the case studies and consider their implications for the development of successful negotiation strategies.

Grant awarding bodies

A key challenge for both neophyte and established researchers is to secure resources to support their research. This entails the development and construction of a formal proposal to be considered for funding in what is typically a highly competitive process. Within the higher education and health service sectors, resources are made available to support different initiatives for which researchers must bid competitively in an internal competition. Research councils, charities and government agencies, such as the Department of Health, also allocate funds to support projects. These funding streams vary in character. Some may be specifically directed at a key area of concern – such as a particular disease – others may be rather broader – such as the The Health Foundation's 'Leading practice through research' programme, where the key concern is on developing the skills of the researcher rather than the proposed topic. Funding can be commissioned or responsive. In responsive mode, researcher initiated projects which meet the funding body's overall remit will be considered. Commissioned research is more specific; proposals are invited on defined topics, with the research questions and in some instances the method clearly prescribed.

As we have argued in Part I, for a range of reasons nurses have limited access to, and knowledge of, established research funding bodies and there is a dearth of dedicated research funds. Moreover, commissioning bodies receive far more high quality proposals than they can afford to fund, and so for even the most experienced researcher the chances of success are slim. Clearly securing funds to support research activity depends to a considerable extent on producing a well-designed high quality study. There are several texts available which offer advice in putting together a winning proposal (Punch, 2000; Delamont and Atkinson, 2004) and we do not intend to rehearse this guidance here. However, we argue that good science is sometimes not sufficient. There is also a need to focus on the political aspects of the funding process in order to maximize the likelihood of success. In the first of the case studies considered in this chapter, Davina describes her experiences of applying for external funding for an ethnographic study of changing roles and responsibilities at the health and social care interface (Allen *et al.*, 2002). She examines how, through a range of negotiation processes, the team designed a research proposal which met the needs of academics, practitioners and policy makers.

From 'The changing shape of nursing practice' to 'Delivering health and social care' – Davina

When I joined the Cardiff School of Nursing and Midwifery Studies shortly after completing my PhD an important objective was to plan a future programme of research which built on the thesis and would attract external funding. This was part of a wider school strategy which stressed the importance of programmatic activity at the individual and departmental level. As we have seen, the policy and service driven nature of funding opportunities can make it very difficult for researchers to sustain a single line of scientific enquiry over several years. However, it was also the case that the University had pump-primed nursing research within the School, with the very explicit expectation that we would lever in external resources. The challenge then was to produce a research plan which was driven by scientific questions, but which would also attract external funding. At this time, the Wales Office for Research and Development (WORD) ran both responsive and commissioned funding streams, and we knew that the next round of responsive grants was imminent.

As the first step towards developing a proposal for submission to WORD, I began by writing a paper which explored different options for future research. This is what Punch (2000) refers to as an 'ideas paper', and others have termed a 'preliminary discussion paper' or a 'discussion and concept paper' (Gilpatrick, 1989). My PhD study was informed by sociological theories of the division of labour and was an ethnographic study of the routine constitution of nursing jurisdiction. The research examined in detail the fine-grained 'boundary work' through which five key nursing interfaces were constructed: nurse–nurse, nurse–doctor, nurse–manager, nurse–patient/family, nurse–health care assistant (Allen, 2001). My interest was in the consequences of these workplace negotiations for the content of nursing work, but as a new post-doctoral researcher I was left with a burning desire to develop further my thinking and examine some of these key interfaces in more detail using the same theoretical framework. Of particular interest was the nurse–patient/family interface. As is typical in ethnography, the focus of the research had shifted over the course of data collection, and this interface was one example of a theme which was not included in the original study design. For this reason, I had not received ethical approval to interview patients and their family carers and, as a consequence, my analysis had to be based on observations on the ward and interviews with nurses. Whilst this was perfectly adequate for the objectives of the thesis, intellectually it felt like unfinished business. Accordingly, my ideas paper was, to a considerable extent, focused on this area of concern. I suggested three linked studies all using an in-depth ethnographic approach, which could be taken forward sequentially.

The 'ideas paper' was used as the basis for discussion with colleagues, who acted as advisors and critical friends. Punch (2000) underlines the value of such discussions, pointing out that the final proposal should be a stand alone document which can be understood by a mixed readership of experts and non-experts and so there is value in making and taking opportunities to discuss ideas. Beyond this, for those unfamiliar with a funding body, sharing work with others who have such a familiarity and preferably have been successful in securing funding, can be most beneficial. This was true in the case of our critical friends who, whilst expressing enthusiasm for pursuing the intellectual lines of enquiry identified, advised us strongly to focus the work around those issues which had immediate policy relevance. They also suggested that we enter into informal discussion with WORD which they indicated was open to the discussion of developing ideas with researchers. This was valuable advice and based on useful intelligence.

As a result of our dialogue with the members of the funding body, it became clear that the priority issue for policy makers and research commissioners was joint working at the health/social care interface. Although we intended applying for responsive mode funding, we took the view that we would increase our likelihood of success if our interests could be dovetailed with those of policy makers. We therefore reoriented our thinking to resonate with these policy concerns, and focused the study much more specifically on management of the health and social care interface. A full proposal was developed (see Figure 7.1), which built on our ideas paper to develop a research design founded on in-depth ethnographic case studies of how the system of health and social care was negotiated around patient need.

We enrolled the support of an impressive range of health and social care providers as co-collaborators on the project. This was very resource intensive but we were fortunate enough to have sufficient time to establish these relationships before the proposal was submitted. This served the purpose of under-writing the perceived relevance of the proposal to practitioners and policy makers, and gave a strong indication that the necessary access to the proposed study sites was secured. We also reasoned that the majority of the members of the commissioning panel were unlikely to be familiar with ethnographic research. Therefore care was taken to avoid the use of jargon and to translate concepts – familiar to a qualitative research audience – into terms which would be understandable to those more familiar with other research paradigms.

The proposal was sent by the funding body for peer review before a decision was reached by the Commissioning Board. At the time, it was the practice of the latter to share reviewers' comments with researchers and permit them an opportunity to respond before a final decision about funding was reached. We were required to formulate our response within a tight timeframe and limit it to a single side of A4.

Figure 7.1 Extract from Project Proposal

Interagency collaboration between health and social services is a well-established concern. Today's carers face additional pressures. Policy developments and health trends have transformed the environment of the caring community creating changes in roles and responsibilities. Service providers face formidable challenges in managing their work boundaries in order to deliver 'seamless' services. Traditionally, governments have looked for structural answers to the problems of service co-ordination. Now the onus has shifted to providers to find local solutions. Our existing knowledge of the impact of these trends is limited. There is, therefore, a need for research to increase understanding of the important features of the interface between health and social care in order to inform the development of roles and responsibilities in the agencies concerned.

The division of labour in society has concerned sociologists for a long time. Drawing on interactionist theories of work, this project will employ a series of ethnographic case studies to explore in-depth changing roles, relationships and working practices in the delivery of health and social care. Adults under-going neurological rehabilitation will be taken as an exemplar group. Six case studies (each of three months duration) will be undertaken at each site, spanning the patient's progress from acute to community care. Comparative data will be collected in three local authorities in separate Welsh health authorities utilizing the following research tools: a mapping exercise of the web of care surrounding the case study subjects, semi-structured interviews with service providers, clients and users, field observations, tape-recordings of meetings and documentary analysis.

There is some evidence to suggest that nurse researchers are very easily crushed by critical reviewers' comments and do not take the opportunity to defend their work or clarify their proposal (Mead *et al.*, 1997). In our case, both reviewers raised concerns about whether the study was adding to new knowledge and whether it represented value for money. We knew from our experience that in the competitive world of research funding, either of these criticisms on its own would be enough to rule a proposal out of the competition at an early stage. Yet we disagreed with both of these concerns, and mounted a robust response. The main threads of our argument were as follows:

I   WORD and service colleagues were widely consulted in the developmental stages of this work and the question of the study's focus was never raised. On the contrary, it was seen as an important area for investigation and the project has received whole-hearted support from health and social services practitioners and managers in the three study sites.

2   That the referees had failed to acknowledge what was different about our proposal and we welcomed the opportunity to make this more explicit. Thus we drew attention to the following: that the work was client focused, specifically concerned with changing roles and relationships and that our theoretical framework – a division of labour perspective – led us to ask different questions from those which had shaped earlier studies.

3   The project had received whole-hearted support from health and social services practitioners and managers in the three study sites. 'There is clearly a felt need for this study in Wales. The support that has been shown for this study from those working at the "sharp end" has been truly overwhelming. We would very much welcome the opportunity to take this work forward'.

Such arguments were clearly partly successful, as an offer was made to fund the work. However, concerns were raised about the costs of the original study and we were encouraged to scale-down our aspirations and re-couch the proposal as pilot research. This we did, by limiting the study to two sites only and focusing specifically on adults who had suffered a first acute stroke. However, because we did not want to compromise the quality of the work and our ability to address the scientific questions which were of interest to us, we elected to part fund the work from internal sources. We originally requested funding of £196,567; we were finally awarded £72,000. Having secured part-funding for the proposal, the next hurdle was to gain ethical approval to undertake the research.

Ethics and research governance committees

The UK has a number of governance frameworks outlining the key responsibilities of all stakeholders involved in health and social care research (Department of Health, 2001; Scottish Executive Health Department, 2001; Wales Office of Research and Development for Health and Social Care, 2001). The Department of Health maintains that the primary consideration in studies should be the dignity, rights, safety and well-being of research participants, and that National Health Service (NHS) research ethics committees (RECs) have a key role to play in this area (Department of Health, 2001). RECs are independent bodies within the NHS, which exist to provide advice on the ethical dimensions of research projects that plan to involve users of health services, carers of health service patients, or NHS staff. They address a wide range of issues, including: the scientific basis of studies; the potential of studies to damage the health of participants; the likelihood and degree of distress and discomfort to participants; and the proposed procedures for obtaining and recording informed consent. In addition, it is usual for RECs to pay particular attention to research studies which aim to include vulnerable patients, including: children; women who may be pregnant; prisoners; and people with mental illnesses or learning disabilities (Tierney, 1995).

In the UK certainly, there is some ambivalence within the research community about health and social care research governance arrangements. Some claim that past experience indicates a clear need for robust regulatory frameworks in order to ensure that research subjects are protected and that health and social care research is of a high quality (Pirohamed, 2002). There are others, however, who have expressed concern that they place unreasonable demands on researchers and that their over-enthusiastic application results in unnecessary bureaucratic complexity that will compound existing demands on the research community. We draw on our experiences of applying for research ethics committee approval for two studies with the same research design in order to explore a number of issues of significance to researchers preparing to navigate a path through this key gate-keeping committee.

A tale of two studies: 'Delivering health and social care' and 'Health and social care for people with severe mental health problems' – Davina and Ben

Over the last decade, the School of Nursing and Midwifery Studies has developed a team-based research strategy focused on broad themes and/or programmes of work with strong research leadership. One such programme of research centres on the organization and delivery of health and social care in which the *Delivering Health and Social Care* (Study 1) project was the first externally funded project. *Health and Social Care for People with Severe Mental Health Problems* (Study 2) replicated the design and broad theoretical framework of Study 1.

Both projects employed a multiple case study, cross-site comparative design. Study 1 focused on adults undergoing stroke rehabilitation, who, in the opinion of service providers, had complex continuing care needs. Four ethnographic case studies were carried out in each of two Welsh health authorities centred on the client and their surrounding web of care. Snowball sampling was used to identify the key players involved in the planning and provision of services in each case. Interviews were carried out with clients and their significant others, and with service providers involved in their care and other key personnel. Critical events, such as case conferences and home visits, were observed and in some instances tape-recorded. Case notes and additional documentation were also consulted. These data were used to build up a comprehensive picture of each case in which their care was mapped.

Study 2 replicated the design of Study 1 but focused on service provision to people with severe mental health problems. Replication studies are valuable in that they permit findings to be compared and contrasted, and encourage the development of methodological expertise within research units. There are also practical benefits as protocols and templates can be shared; both the information sheets produced for Study 2, and applications submitted for REC approval, drew heavily on documents produced in Study 1.

Applying for ethical approval

In Study 1 it was necessary to apply to two RECs because the research was being carried out in two health authorities. In both cases REC approval was granted in a straightforward way. However, despite the fact that it drew heavily on the research design used in Study 1 and utilized the template for the REC application form, the experience of obtaining REC approval in Study 2 was very different.

Unlike Study 1 which was focused on adults who had suffered a stroke, Study 2 planned to include people with mental health difficulties. It is usual to regard people experiencing mental health problems as being particularly vulnerable research participants (Koivisto et al., 2001). People with major mental illnesses such as schizophrenia are often considered to lack the capacity needed to give their informed consent to participate in research studies. 'Capacity' in this context refers to the ability of individuals to exercise autonomy and self-determination (Drane, 1984).

One approach is to exclude all those with 'impairment or disturbance of mental functioning' from participating in research studies. However, this would result in the unnecessary protection of individuals who, whilst experiencing some degree of mental impairment or disturbance, also possess the ability to give consent (Usher and Holmes, 1997) and would lead to their views and experiences remaining unknown. Moreover, an individual's 'capacity' is not an absolute; the ability to exercise autonomy and to make informed decisions – for all people, and not just those with mental health difficulties – can fluctuate.

An additional ethical dimension was raised by the decision to include in the research sample people whose care and treatment was organized under sections of the Mental Health Act (1983) for England and Wales. The Act establishes the conditions under, and the procedures through which people with mental disorders can be compulsorily admitted to hospital for the purposes of assessment and treatment. The Act also sets out the broad principles for the provision of 'aftercare'. The inclusion in research studies of people subject to sections of the Mental Health Act needs to be done with extreme care. People whose care and treatment is organized under sections of the Act are under a form of constraint. This places an additional obligation on researchers to ensure that those who participate in studies give 'true' informed consent (Wing, 1999). Guidance on the inclusion in studies of detained patients does exist, but seems contradictory.

The initial application for REC approval in the second study stressed awareness of the range of ethical issues raised by the proposal. Criteria for the selection of case study subjects were also included, as Figure 7.2 shows.

This initial REC application was unsuccessful. The REC had a number of concerns with the application for ethical approval. First, the committee considered that the objectives in Study 2 could not be met. Yet in Study 1 two successful REC applications were made which described the same objectives and the same research methods. The committee did not elaborate upon its conclusions and so the reasons for its decision remain opaque. However, this does raise the issue of consistency in research governance processes (see for example Nicholl, 2000).

One possible explanation for the inconsistency could have been their differing degrees of understanding of qualitative methods, and of the value of undertaking qualitative studies. There is literature indicating that RECs sometimes fail to understand research which proposes to use non-quantitative methods (see for

Figure 7.2 Extracts from first application for research ethics committee approval in Study 2

The aims and objectives of this study determine that access be gained to individuals whose difficulties are both severe and long-lasting. Access may, therefore, be sought to individuals who are subject to sections of the Mental Health Act (1983) at their point of entry into the study. Access may also be sought to individuals who remain subject to formal care and treatment throughout the duration of their participation in the project. This would include, for example, the case of an individual discharged from hospital to home under Section 25 of the Mental Health (Patients in the Community) Act (1995). Finally, there is the possibility that some individuals may become subject to the provisions of the Act during their participation in the study.

In seeking ethical approval to include people detained under the Act in this study, the following criteria for their participation are offered. First, no individuals suffering from an acute episode of mental illness will be approached in order to request their participation in the project. Hospital inpatients detained under the Act will only be approached as they are preparing for discharge into the community. Second, in the case of individuals subject to sections of the Act and approaching hospital discharge, the assent of the nearest relative and/or significant other will be sought. This will be in addition to the seeking of the informed consent of the service user him/herself. Third, where an individual participating in the study becomes acutely ill and is admitted to hospital, either informally or, particularly, under a section of the Mental Health Act, the assent of the nearest relative and/or significant other to the continued following of the service user's care will be sought. In all instances, the assent of appropriate clinicians, the Responsible Medical Officer [consultant psychiatrist] included, will also be sought. No extra demands will be made on either service users or their informal carers during critical periods, such as those associated with admission to hospital. Practitioners will also be asked, where appropriate, to give only retrospective accounts of their work during the period after caring for an acutely ill case study subject.

It is, finally, anticipated that the background of the principal researcher as a qualified and experienced community mental health nurse will be invaluable in ensuring that the clinical needs of case study subjects remain paramount, and in ensuring that professional judgement and sensitivity is maintained throughout the period in which all service users participate in the study.

example Dolan, 1999; Gelling, 1999; Stevenson and Beech, 1998). Dolan (1999) has argued that limited knowledge of qualitative research by RECs presents itself as a particular problem for nurse researchers, who may be more likely than other health researchers to design studies which use non-quantitative methods.

The studies also had differences which may have helped to shape the committees' decisions. At the time the REC applications were made, Study 1 had already received external research funding and this may have functioned to afford it a legitimacy in the eyes of the committee compared to Study 2, which at that point had no external funding. Moreover, it was a requirement of the REC application forms to state whether the research was being undertaken as part of a programme of study. Whilst Study 1 was undertaken by an experienced research team, Study 2 was being carried out for the purposes of a PhD, and this may have resulted in the committee taking a more critical stance. REC decision-making inevitably takes place in a social context, and members deploy a number of processes in order to find meaning in a given situation (Garfinkel, 1967). Although we cannot say with any certainty how significant these key differences between the two studies were in practice, it has raised our awareness of the subtle clues that are contained in application forms, and has heightened our sensitivity to issues of interpretation and presentation.

The resubmitted application for ethical approval in Study 2 was designed to address the committee's concerns (Figure 7.3). The study objectives were condensed with the aim of improving clarity, and the relationship between Study 1 and Study 2 was more strongly emphasized. In addition, the long tradition of ethnographic research and its capacity to generate important data associated with the provision of health and social care was underlined.

The second objection raised by the REC related to issues of access. The REC criticized the application for having insufficient detail about service providers who would be involved in the study. It also noted that it was unclear who would assess the 'fitness' of patients to participate in the project. These objections raise further research governance issues: first, the relationship between seeking REC approval and negotiating access to study sites. In Study 2, the view of the ethics committee appeared to be that access negotiations should have started before an application was made for ethical approval. However, as later experience in Study 2 demonstrated, one of the first questions which health and social care 'gatekeepers' typically ask during access negotiations in research sites is whether formal ethical approval has been obtained. In Study 1 it was a requirement of the application for research funding that key research collaborators were identified, and service managers, senior clinicians and policy makers had agreed to support the study and function as a steering group. Whilst none were in a position to grant direct access to the study sites in which the research was taken forward, the identification of key service collaborators appears to have satisfied both RECs.

The REC's response to the second study proposal also raises important questions regarding the control of research access to health service users. The committee in this case stated that only a medical practitioner could assess the capacity of individual patients to give informed consent. This statement granted a powerful research 'gatekeeping' role to members of the medical profession (Service Users' Experiences

Figure 7.3 Extracts from second application for research ethics committee approval in Study 2

The final report arising from [Study 1] has been favourably received, and has demonstrated the value of in-depth qualitative research methods as a means of generating answers to important questions associated with the provision of health and social care.

Principal objectives for this study are to:

1   investigate the ways in which health and social care professionals manage their respective roles and responsibilities in the delivery of services to eight case study subjects with severe mental health problems;
2   map the network of health and social care providers involved in each of the case study subjects over a four-month period;
3   identify the factors which, in the opinion of local stakeholders, contribute to or detract from the effectiveness of interagency and interprofessional collaboration in the study settings;
4   locate the research findings within the local and national policy context.

Subjects will be purposively selected in consultation with the responsible consultant psychiatrists and with other health and social care professionals. One criterion for subject selection will be the responsible consultant's assessment of the capacity of identified clients to give informed consent. The enclosed letters from [two consultant psychiatrists] indicate that they have agreed to take on this responsibility. Once potential subjects have been identified, the initial invitation to participate will be made on behalf of the principal researcher by appropriately placed practitioners.

The aims and objectives of the study determine that access may be sought to individuals who are subject to sections of the Mental Health Act (1983). How care is delivered to people whose care and treatment is organized under sections of the Act is of particular analytic interest. Providing aftercare services under Section 117, for example, is a critical test of the ability of different professionals and agencies to collaborate effectively. It is of equal analytic interest to gain an understanding of how well services work together when sections of the Mental Health Act are first applied for, and when individuals are formally admitted to hospital. It is also possible that some of the selected subjects may experience episodes of acute mental illness during their participation in the study.

These issues raise important ethical concerns. In the most recent edition of the Mental Health Act Code of Practice (Department of Health and Welsh Office, 1999), it is stated that 'mental disorder does not necessarily make a patient incapable of giving or refusing consent' (Section 15.12). In its position paper on research involving patients detained under the Mental Health Act (1983), moreover, the Mental Health Act Commission (1997) has proposed that, 'if a patient has capacity to consent to

continued...

Figure 7.3 continued...

participation in research, and does in fact give actual and informed consent, then participation should not be prevented unless (a) involvement conflicts with any provision of the 1983 Act; (b) involvement is inconsistent with treatment being received as a detained patient'.

In seeking REC approval to include in this study people detained under the Mental Health Act (1983), and to include people who may experience episodes of acute mental illness during the period of their participation, the following criteria are offered:

Patients approached to participate in the study will only include those who have been assessed by the responsible consultant psychiatrist as having capacity to consent; only patients who have capacity to consent and who actually give informed consent will be included; patients will only enter the study with the explicit agreement of the responsible consultant; no individuals suffering from an acute episode of mental illness will be approached in order to request their participation in the study.

The agreement of the responsible consultant to the continued participation of case study subjects who become acutely ill will be obtained.

Where an individual participating in the study becomes acutely ill, the assent of the nearest relative and/or significant other to the continued following of the service user's care will be sought.

Following guidance from the Mental Health Act Commission (1997), the Approved Social Worker (ASW) and other involved mental health professionals working with detained patients will be consulted prior to an approach being made to the patients to participate in the study.

Hospital inpatients detained under the Act will only be approached to participate as they are preparing for discharge into the community.

In the case of individuals subject to sections of the Act and approaching hospital discharge, in addition to the obtaining of the patient's informed consent the assent of the nearest relative and/or significant other will be sought, subject to the patient's agreement to this approach being made.

Throughout this study, the background of the principal researcher as a qualified and experienced community mental health nurse will be invaluable in ensuring that the clinical needs of case study subjects remain paramount, and in ensuring that professional judgement and sensitivity is maintained.

Research Group School of Nursing and Midwifery Studies University of Wales College of Medicine, 2000), which whilst symptomatic of the power of medical discourse, runs counter to current trends in health and social care delivery in the UK (Department of Health, 1998).

In response to the REC's concerns, access negotiations with key individuals in each of the two selected study sites were brought forward. An important task was to secure letters of support from senior professionals, which were later attached to the resubmitted REC application as evidence of collaboration. Over the course of these negotiations the interdependence of negotiating research access and achieving ethical approval was explicitly discussed with the study participants, who became partners in the process of securing the REC's agreement that Study 2 could proceed.

Considerable work was also undertaken to address the REC's concerns regarding the possible inclusion of people subject to sections of the Mental Health Act, and to address the questions raised about the assessment of suitability to take part in the study. The committee stated that it was not clear whether liaison regarding the fitness of detained patients to participate would take place with responsible medical practitioners, or with 'medical officers appointed under the terms of the Mental Health Act'. The REC's suggestion that it might be necessary to obtain the opinion of independent doctors regarding the suitability of people subject to sections of the Act to take part in the study runs contrary to the position of the Mental Health Act Commission (MHAC). The second REC application (Figure 7.3) included information directly extracted from the MHAC's position paper on research involving detained patients (Mental Health Act Commission, 1997). Material was also included from the current Mental Health Act Code of Practice (Department of Health and Welsh Office, 1999). The new application also included explicit information about the selection of service users to take part in the study, the assessment of their suitability, and the processes through which they would be recruited.

Unexpected outcomes

This new REC application was submitted to the same panel that had scrutinized, and rejected, the first application. Their response was most unexpected: the committee wrote that it had '... agreed that your proposal was a survey and as such was outside the remit of the research ethics committee'. This was a surprising outcome, given the range of questions raised by the panel in its first deliberation. Many of the issues identified in the first application had been addressed in the resubmitted proposal; nonetheless, it was still not expected to hear that the planned research was, from the REC's perspective, either not 'research' at all, or not 'research' which required REC approval. At a pragmatic level this decision meant that the study could proceed. The approach taken to the recruitment of case study subjects followed the procedure detailed in the resubmitted REC application, and reproduced in Figure 7.3. We took the view that the responsibility to ensure that studies are ethically sound lies with the researchers. Preparing research proposals for formal ethical scrutiny is an important exercise in obliging researchers to think critically about the ethical dimensions of their studies. Whatever the outcome of an application to a REC, however, the ethical dilemmas raised in the day-to-day undertaking of a research project can only be addressed by the researcher or the research team.

Discussion

So what are the learning points to be gleaned from our experiences? The over-whelming lesson to be gained from an analysis of the above case studies is that gate-keeping committees are comprised of people. Despite the existence of criteria and protocols to guide decision making, it is inevitable that a committee's work will be the product of the interaction of the individuals which constitute its membership and the diverse experiences, understanding and agenda that they bring to the decision-making processes. This helps to explain some of their well-documented weaknesses which are revealed in our case studies: the lack of standardization between committees in the ways in which they process applications (Redshaw *et al.*, 1996); the inconsistencies in outcome which can be encountered when identical or similar research proposals are scrutinized by different committees (Nicholl, 2000) and the opacity of funding decisions. These issues can be significant problems for health and social care researchers, but it is possible to take some action to avoid common pitfalls.

Understanding the role of the committee

It is clearly essential to understand the role of the relevant committee and the questions, concerns and priorities that are likely to be uppermost in the minds of its members. It is also helpful to understand the committee's business, role and function. For example, an objection that is frequently raised by researchers about the role of RECs is that they go beyond their remit and pass judgement on the methodological basis of studies rather than focusing exclusively on the ethical dimensions (see for example Dolan, 1999). Yet RECs quite rightly argue that they are perfectly entitled to make such assessments as participation in studies which are methodologically flawed and will not be able to meet their objectives is, in their view, unethical. One may wish to argue about the extent to which the membership of committees includes the relevant expertise to make such judgements, but this does not in any way alter RECs' mandate. It it is useful to obtain the criteria the committee works to. This is often in a tick box format to aid decision making. Within the School at Cardiff, we treat intelligence on key gate-keeping committees as a collective resource and maintain a data base of individuals with experience of negotiating with relevant committees and funding bodies who can advise colleagues. Members of staff who have reviewed proposals or have served on commissioning bodies are particular assets as they have an understanding of the inner workings of such groupings. The novice researcher would be advised to seek out such people in order to support the application process.

The composition of committees – knowing your audience

It is also useful to have a sense of the composition of committees so that you can tailor your submission to this audience. It is likely for example, that nurse researchers will be submitting their proposals to committees consisting mainly of members of the medical profession, social scientists or policy makers who may be unfamiliar with nursing research priorities and the methods most appropriate to their study. Furthermore, as we have seen, different groups have different expectations of what research can deliver and it is important that work is appropriately pitched for the audience. Our experiences have revealed evidence of a continued bias towards biomedical science. This was shown in the limited understanding of qualitative research demonstrated by the REC which scrutinized Study 2. Recent efforts have been made to raise awareness within the medical (see for example Pope and Mays, 1995) and the policy-making communities (Murphy *et al.*, 1998) about the contribution which qualitative studies can make, but it may still be necessary to engage in a process of 'translation' when presenting work to bodies which are more familiar with other methods and/or disciplines.

Building relationships and seeking expert advice

Our case studies also illustrate the importance of building relationships and seeking expert advice. We have shown how, in the example of applying for research funding, talking to people who were more familiar with the commissioning body to which we intended applying was instrumental in shaping the final direction of the study. Both case studies, like those described by Nicola and Linda in Chapter 6, also underline the importance of making contact with the people concerned and entering into dialogue with them to build shared understanding. We cannot be certain about what factors were most significant in our successful application for funding, given the criticisms raised by both referees. However, having established a dialogue with WORD representatives and service providers, we could point to their support for a study of this particular kind. Had these conversations not occurred we would have been without this strong line of defence.

Planning and sequencing

Our case studies have also shown the importance of sequencing. It is important to plan carefully and be very clear about what needs to be done and in what order. This was clearly demonstrated in our consideration of the research ethics application in Study 2. After the rejection of the first application, the processes of applying for ethical approval and negotiating access to study sites became closely interwoven. Sufficient time should be allocated to develop the proposal so that crucial deadlines are not missed.

Presentation of the work

In negotiating a path through a key gate-keeping committee, one should be aware that its members are ordinarily volunteers who undertake this work in addition to their normal responsibilities. Remember that yours will be one of a large number of applications being considered. Delamont and Atkinson (2004) argue that 'one should assume [...] that anyone reading the application has insufficient time to devote to the task, has multiple calls on their attention, and would rather be doing something more enjoyable'. Every effort therefore should be made to ensure that the application is clearly presented and ideas expressed with clarity and precision. Key information should be immediately apparent and '[W]hile grants are not awarded on the basis of artistic impression – unlike figure skating – anything that can distract or antagonize the reviewers should be avoided' (Delamont and Atkinson, 2004). Moreover, as we have seen there is also a need to be sensitive to the interpretative work that inevitably goes on in decision making, and ensure that the information contained in applications is unequivocal.

Grant-awarding bodies and research governance and ethics committees increasingly require applicants to attend meetings and defend their work. This was the case in Study 2, where an (eventually successful) application for funding to the Smith and Nephew Foundation led to an invitation to attend a panel meeting in which the merits of the proposal would be discussed. Such occasions should be treated rather like a job interview, with careful prior preparation and consideration of the presentation of self. If you are required to give a formal presentation of your work – which was not required when Study 2 was considered by the Smith and Nephew Foundation panel – give this the same attention you would a conference presentation. Think about your audience, and practise beforehand to ensure that you keep to the allocated time and try to anticipate possible questions.

Balancing confidence with concession

Mead *et al.* (1997) point to the importance of stamina in pursuing a research proposal to a successful conclusion and this holds true for most gate-keeping committees. These authors observe that nurse researchers often drop out of the peer review process by failing to respond to referees' comments. It is regrettably true that referees' comments can often be very critical and it can be difficult for even the most experienced researcher to remain unaffected by this, but it is important to persevere. Referees' comments should be considered carefully and probing questions asked as to their validity. If a referee has made an important point which should be addressed then it is sensible to acknowledge this. It is possible to disagree with the referee's comments, in which case there is a need to mount a carefully worded and convincing defence. The trick is to balance confidence with concession.

Conclusion

Good ideas, good science and proper attention to the ethical dimensions of studies are necessary components of all research proposals. They are not always sufficient, however, in persuading powerful gatekeepers to give their blessing to studies. Knowing that the deliberations of grant awarding, ethical scrutiny and NHS trust bodies are contextualized, interactive processes helps researchers tailor their proposals accordingly. Novice researchers can help themselves by tapping into the accumulated intelligence relating to gate-keeping committees which more experienced colleagues are likely to possess. In all cases it is particularly useful to remember that committees are likely to be peopled by time-pressed individuals with multiple calls on their expertise. Holding this in mind makes for research proposals which are unambiguously and succinctly worded, and suitably 'translated' for their intended audiences. Attending to the politics and presentation of research proposals in this way brings no guarantee of success with gate-keeping bodies, but does at least maximize the chances of hurdles of this type being successfully negotiated.

Acknowledgements

Study 1 was partially supported through a grant from the Wales Office of Research and Development for Health and Social Care, and Study 2 was partially supported through the award of a Nursing Research Fellowship from the Smith and Nephew Foundation. This chapter draws substantially on a previously published manuscript: Hannigan, B. and Allen, D. (2003) 'A tale of two studies: observations on research governance issues arising from studies of complex caring interfaces', *Journal of International Nursing Studies*, 40(7): 685–95, which is reproduced with permission from Elsevier.

References

Allen, D. (2001) *The Changing Shape of Nursing Practice: The Role of Nurses in the Hospital Division of Labour*, London: Routledge.

Allen, D., Lyne, P. and Griffiths, L. (2002) 'Studying complex caring interfaces: key issues arising from a study of multi-agency rehabilitative care for people who have suffered a stroke', *Journal of Clinical Nursing*, 11, 297–305.

Delamont, S. and Atkinson, P. (2004) *Successful Research Careers: A Practical Guide*, Buckingham: Open University Press.

Department of Health (1998) *A First Class Service: Quality in the New NHS*, London: Department of Health.

—— (2001) *Research Governance Framework for Health and Social Care*, London, Department of Health.

Department of Health and Welsh Office (1999) *Code of Practice: Mental Health Act 1983*, London: The Stationery Office.

Dolan, B. (1999) Guest editorial: 'The impact of local research ethics committees on the development of nursing knowledge', *Journal of Advanced Nursing*, 30, 1009–10.

Drane, J.F. (1984) 'Competency to give an informed consent: a model for making clinical assessments', *Journal of the American Medical Association*, 252, 925–7.

Garfinkel, H. (1967) *Studies in Ethnomethodology*, Englewood Cliffs, NJ: Prentice Hall.

Gelling, L. (1999) 'Role of the research ethics committee', *Nurse Education Today*, 19, 564–9.

Gilpatrick, E. (1989) *Grants for Nonprofit Organizations: A Guide to Funding and Grant Writing*, New York: Praeger.

Koivisto, K., Janhonen, S., Latvala, E. and Väisänen, L. (2001) 'Applying ethical guidelines in nursing research on people with mental illness', *Nursing Ethics*, 8, 328–39.

Mead, D., Moseley, L. and Cook, R. (1997) 'The performance of nursing in the research stakes: lessons from the field', *Nursing Times Research*, 2, 335–44.

Mental Health Act Commission (1997) *Research Involving Detained Patients*, Nottingham: Mental Health Act Commission.

Murphy, E., Dingwall, R., Greatbatch, D., Parker, S. and Watson, P. (1998) *Qualitative Research Methods in Health Technology Assessment: A Review of the Literature*, London: Health Technology Assessment.

Nicholl, J. (2000) 'The ethics of research ethics committees', *British Medical Journal*, 320, 1217.

Pirohamed, J. (2002) 'Informed consent in clinical research – are we doing it properly?', Annual RCN Research Society Conference. University of Exeter, Exeter.

Pope, C. and Mays, N. (1995) 'Qualitative research: reaching the parts others methods cannot reach: an introduction to qualitative methods in health and health services research', *British Medical Journal*, 311, 42–5.

Punch, K.F. (2000) *Developing Effective Research Proposals*, London: Sage.

Redshaw, M.A., Harris, A. and Baum, J.D. (1996) 'Research ethics committee audit: differences between committees', *Journal of Medical Ethics*, 22, 78–82.

Scottish Executive Health Department (2001) *Research Governance Framework for Health and Community Care*, Edinburgh: Scottish Executive.

Service Users' Experiences Research Group School of Nursing and Midwifery Studies University of Wales College of Medicine (2000) *User Involvement in User-focused Research* [Working Paper 1], Cardiff, School of Nursing and Midwifery Studies, University of Wales College of Medicine.

Stevenson, C. and Beech, I. (1998) 'Playing the power game for qualitative researchers: the possibility of a post-modern approach', *Journal of Advanced Nursing*, 27, 790–7.

Tierney, A. (1995) 'The role of research ethics committees', *Nurse Researcher*, 3, 43–52.

Usher, K. and Holmes, C. (1997) 'Ethical aspects of phenomenological research with mentally ill people', *Nursing Ethics*, 4, 49–56.

Wales Office of Research and Development for Health and Social Care (2001) *Research Governance Framework for Health and Social Care in Wales*, Cardiff: Wales Office of Research and Development for Health and Social Care.

Wing, J. (1999) 'Ethics and psychiatry research', in S. Bloch, P. Chodoff and S.A. Green (eds) *Psychiatric Ethics*, 3rd edn, Oxford: Oxford University Press.

Chapter 8

Data generation

Ben Hannigan

Introduction

This chapter is the first of two to examine the relationship between nurse researchers and their data. Underpinning this contribution is the idea that research data are never simply 'out there' waiting to be casually picked up by the passing investigator. Instead, the work required of researchers in this phase of their studies is usefully captured by the phrase 'data generation', which hints at the purposeful activity in which researchers engage. In contrast, a term like 'data collection' misleads by implying that – like leaves on an autumn day – data found 'lying about' can simply be swept up.

In some nursing research textbooks discussion of data generation issues is limited to a review of techniques, such as the characteristics of methods of data creation. Technical, or toolkit, accounts risk understating the importance of reflexivity in the conduct of both qualitative and quantitative studies. Reflexivity refers to an active awareness of the circumstances in, and the practicalities through which, data are produced (Allen, 2004). A reflexive stance also acknowledges the significance of the researcher's values, attitudes and other aspects of personal and professional biography in shaping the character of the data produced.

The case studies

The first case study drawn on in this chapter is the *All Wales Community Mental Health Nursing Stress Study* (subsequently referred to as the Stress Study). This began in 1998, with a final report appearing in 2001. Research team members, myself included, were able to refer to personal practitioner experiences to confirm the personal challenges associated with work in community care settings. Our experiences, and previous research, pointed towards rising workloads, upwardly spiralling administrative responsibilities and inadequate resourcing as sources of stress.

The second study drawn on in this chapter – *Health and Social Care for People with Severe Mental Health Problems* (referred to in this case study as Health and Social Care) – is an ongoing investigation into the organization and delivery of community care. This project is also a case study for Chapter 7, where further details can be found.

Identifying and generating types of data

One approach to data creation emphasizes the logical relationships between data generation and a study's aims, objectives and theoretical underpinnings. Research aims and theoretical frameworks do not always need to be developed from scratch; indeed, in mature research-led disciplines knowledge typically accumulates incrementally, with studies carefully and explicitly building on what has gone before. Experienced scholars will often think and act as members of a wider research community, networking with colleagues in the shared pursuit of knowledge. Nurses, particularly novice nurse researchers, sometimes lack the confidence to act in this way, and may for example shy away from making contact with established investigators.

In the Stress Study one of our first activities was to make contact with the principal researcher of the Claybury Study (Carson and Kuipers, 1998), Jerome Carson from London's Institute of Psychiatry. This had hitherto been the UK's largest investigation into stress and burnout in community mental health nurses (CMHNs) and there were theoretical and methodological lessons to be learnt from this contact. For example, in our study we decided to follow Carson and his collaborators by adopting a three-tier conceptual model of the stress process (Carson and Kuipers, 1998). This derives from the discipline of psychology, and recognizes that both personal and environmental factors have a bearing on stress. Stressors are viewed as arising from three main sources: work itself, significant life events, and personal aggravations and uplifts. The second element in the framework includes mediating factors, which include self-esteem, personal control, and emotional stability. The model's final element is stress outcomes. Positive outcomes include high levels of job satisfaction, whilst poor outcomes include psychological ill health, low job satisfaction and burnout.

Our adoption of a three-tier model influenced both our overarching objectives and our identification of the types of data we needed to create. Our objectives for the study were to: examine the variety, frequency and severity of stressors experienced by CMHNs; describe the coping strategies used by CMHNs to reduce work-based stress and determine stress outcomes.

Our 'types of data' deliberations were also shaped by our knowledge of the data generation strategies employed in previous investigations. Surveying what is known in a field of study is an essential part of the research endeavour, and reviewing the stress and nursing literature was another of our earliest activities. The fruits of this work were contained in the first publication arising from this study (Edwards *et al.*, 2000). In addition to getting us started our review sharpened our methodological thinking. We unearthed shortcomings in previous research, in both choice of data generation methods and selection of data sources. Previous investigators had tended to use relatively small samples, and to have recruited participants from limited geographical areas. Whilst survey methods were the most widely used means of generating data, many earlier researchers had elected to devise their own questionnaires.

Constructing one-off, tailored, measures offers researchers the opportunity to play an active part in shaping the character of the data to be generated. However, the use of novel measures in quantitative research may also reveal a misunderstanding of the incremental way in which scholarship progresses; novice researchers may assume that only original tools are able to produce original contributions to knowledge. New tools may lack desirable measurement properties. In a field such as stress research, a team may seek to compare its countable data with data generated in related studies with the aim of identifying possible trends. Comparisons of this type are hindered by the use of multiple measures to 'count' similar phenomena.

Measuring tools do not select themselves, and a reflexive stance to the identification and presentation of instruments is warranted. Each researcher needs to develop awareness of the assumptions which they make about the desired properties of their selected instruments, the meaning of the data generated by their use and the consequences arising from any limitations inherent in the toolkit which they finally employ. Standard research texts in nursing set out desiderata such as the various types of reliability and validity, but rarely deal with the question of determining what is 'good enough' for the achievement of the aims of a particular study, given its context. In our case, the key requirements were that the instruments should be suitable for self-completion by our respondents (CMNHs) and should have construct validity in relation to the elements of the theoretical model under investigation. Our methodological decision making was assisted by our success in securing funding from the General Nursing Council for England and Wales Trust, which allowed us to consider the use of commercially available tools.

In making our final research instrument selections we therefore took care to choose measures sensitive to the generation of data consistent with our stress model. The only tool devised solely for the study was the 19-item Welsh CMHN Stress Study Demographic Questionnaire. We knew from both practitioner experience and from knowledge of the characteristics of the workforce (Brooker and White, 1997) that CMHNs are a heterogeneous group, and can be found working with a wide variety of service users in a number of different settings. The organizational context in which CMHNs work also varies. In this tool we therefore asked questions relating to issues such as caseload size, client group specialization and team location – all issues which we suspected might be significantly associated with experiences of stress and its consequences.

To measure stressors, we used the CMHN Stress Questionnaire (Revised) (Brown et al., 1995). This previously validated tool was developed in the Claybury Study specifically for use with samples of mental health nurses, and includes questions relating to a wide range of stress-inducing factors which we recognized as being peculiar to the work of CMHNs. For example, we knew that stressors for community mental health practitioners can include the lack of additional resources, and the existence of long waiting lists for access to particular services such as those provided by clinical psychologists. In including questions directed at these and related areas, this questionnaire demonstrated a degree of sensitivity to the context in which CMHNs work.

Stress moderators were measured using two tools: the relatively new PsychNurse Methods of Coping Questionnaire (McElfatrick et al., 2000), which gives information on six types of coping strategy, and the Rosenberg Self Attitude Scale (Rosenberg, 1985) modified by (Wycherley, 1987). The PsychNurse Questionnaire was recommended by Jerome Carson, and our study helped to further test the properties of this measure. Finally, we selected two internationally used measures for the generation of stress outcome data: the 12-item version of the General Health Questionnaire (Goldberg and Williams, 1988), and the Maslach Burnout Inventory (Maslach et al., 1996). These two measures were available to us only through our acquisition of external funding; permission to use a measure always needs to be obtained from its copyright holder. This process can sometimes cost money. In our case, the time taken in selecting – and paying for – the best available tools represented effort and resources well-spent.

In identifying potential sources of data we cast a wide net, and made the early decision to undertake a total population study of all CMHNs working in Wales. This decision was informed by findings from the then current fourth quinquennial community mental health nursing survey for England and Wales (Brooker and White, 1997). From this we knew that an all-Wales investigation was achievable in both resource and feasibility terms.

In this chapter's second case study, *Health and Social Care for People with Severe Mental Health Problems*, community mental health care is theorized as being a dynamic system of work (Hughes, 1971; Abbott, 1988). This theoretical framework also sees work as being, at root, a process of social interaction (Hughes, 1971; Freidson, 1976). This 'ecological' stance has a long tradition in the discipline of sociology, and was also an approach which had been used to underpin earlier projects undertaken in the School of Nursing and Midwifery Studies in Cardiff – including in a study from which I planned to replicate my design and methods. Selection of a theoretical framework needs to be done reflexively. In this case my working knowledge of mental health care as a complex and interrelated system, in which multiple groups and agencies have a part to play, made for a high degree of 'fit' between an ecological approach and my practice-derived experiences.

Adoption of this theoretical stance had major implications for the study's objectives (see Chapter 7 and Figure 8.2 below) and for methodological decision-making. Health and Social Care's design was based on a series of ethnographic case studies. Case study research is well-suited as a means of improving understanding of organizations, and of generating knowledge in conditions where the researcher has little or no control over the behaviours and events under investigation (Yin, 1994; Ferlie, 2001). Each 'case' was an individual user of community mental health services and his or her network of care, set in the organizational context of the wider health and social care setting within which it was located. Having obtained the agreement of service users to participate, in each case study snowball sampling was used to identify the range of professionals, paraprofessionals and informal carers involved in providing services. Initial contact was made with one or more key informants (such as a community mental health nurse), with each being used to put me in touch with further informants. In each of the six case studies this process continued until all those providing significant care had been identified. Data were generated using in-depth qualitative methods. Observational methods were selected for their value in permitting direct access to the everyday, negotiated, division of labour as this was played out in specific workplaces. Protracted, semi-structured interviews were chosen as a means of exploring roles and responsibilities, and of generating data relating to significant but otherwise inaccessible events. A final arm of the data creation strategy was the acquisition and analysis of documents.

Data of the type produced in this study differ substantially from the types of data generated through postal questionnaires; indeed, interview data are different from observational data, which are different again from documentary analysis data (Wolcott, 2001). As we found in the Stress Study, selecting data generation tools for a postal survey is an active process. However, once selections have been made, sources of data identified and access to these negotiated, the survey researcher assumes a lesser role at the point that data are actually generated through the completion and return of questionnaires. In contrast, in ethnographic studies the researcher's role is a particularly active one throughout the totality of the data generation process. A significant investment of 'the self' is called for (for a discussion see Coffey, 1999). The researcher participating in the field *is* the tool of data generation (Hammersley and Atkinson, 1995). Nurses producing ethnographic data can use their practice experiences to inform this process. For example, personal experiences can be actively drawn on during interviews to stimulate discussion, and observational strategies can be refined. However, care also needs to be taken that the researcher's prior familiarity with the field of study does not blind him or her to relevant information, or result in the generation of data which merely confirms deep-rooted preconceptions about the characteristics of the phenomena under investigation.

Identifying and negotiating access to data sources

All researchers, whatever their chosen strategies for data generation, have to work hard to successfully secure access to their data sources (see also Chapter 7). Whilst in the Stress Study we knew the likely size of the total population of CMHNs in Wales this knowledge gave us no insights into how, practically, to contact members of this group. We were aware that seeking access to NHS staff for research purposes is subject to a form of politics. For example, it can speed negotiations to know to whom to address an initial request for institutional access approval. Similarly, lack of familiarity with internal management and professional structures creates the risk that letters requesting research access will disappear into organizational black holes.

As a research team in the Stress Study we were relatively well-connected in some NHS trusts, but less so in others – particularly those more geographically distant from our base. The access strategy we settled on was to first make contact with the chief executives of all Welsh NHS trusts providing community mental health care. We requested permission to approach CMHNs, and asked for the name of a contact person able to help the project's full-time researcher gain access. Our letter also conveyed practical information about our research plans and contained important messages about the research team and our affiliations. Headed paper denoted our status as members of a well-known and respected university. We also demonstrated knowledge of existing research, and presented our plans as part of a wider School strategy. Inevitably, this first letter needed to be followed up in some areas; the urgency felt by us to progress our investigation was not felt in the same way by hard-pressed NHS managers. Many months were needed to negotiate institutional access to all relevant trusts, and to generate a complete list of appropriately-placed contacts able to help us distribute questionnaires.

Through local contacts individual CMHNs were issued with a questionnaire booklet and a return envelope addressed either to the trust contact person or to the dedicated project researcher. The choice of method used to secure the return of questionnaires was agreed between the research team and each trust contact. Therein lay a lesson learnt. Whilst responses were always placed in sealed envelopes before leaving the hands of practitioners, we received feedback from some advising us of their anxieties in returning their questionnaires via a third party. A reflexive stance is demonstrated by the paying of attention to the context in which data are generated, and by learning from this as is appropriate. Thus in our more recent investigation into the association between burnout and clinical supervision, again using CMHNs in Wales as our sample, we opted to receive directly all completed questionnaires using stamped, addressed envelopes and have none passing through intermediaries.

Securing access to sources of data in Health and Social Care was a challenge of a different variety. Institutional access again needed to be negotiated, this time to two NHS trusts and two local authorities. It is useful to know something of the internal politics of organizations to which research access is being sought, and to nurture good relations with well-placed individuals able to champion a research plan. My practitioner experiences were valuable during this period, both in building relationships and in beginning the process of data generation.

One of my earliest access negotiation meetings was held with a senior mental health services manager working in the NHS trust in my first study site. During this event I explicitly drew on my mental health nursing experiences to justify my plans, and to highlight the ways in which findings from my study would be useful to people involved in the provision of care. From my practice experiences I knew that, typically, mental health services can only be developed when NHS and local authority organizations work together. This knowledge helped sensitize me to the significance of some of the comments made by this important gatekeeper on interagency relations in her area. This experience also underlined the degree to which, in addition to negotiating fieldwork access, I was already beginning the process of data generation:

> A very positive meeting, in which I came to realize that I was, as well as negotiating access, also data generating. Denise [manager] [...] is in favour of my project, and has suggested I base myself in the Midtown CMHT. Denise has recently initiated a CMHT management group, which next meets on February 18th. She chairs this group, which is also attended by other key health and social care people. These are, absolutely, the people I need to speak to with respect to access. Denise has promised to put my research on the agenda, and will contact me thereafter. She will also find out what needs to be done with respect to pathways within the trust relating to gaining permission.
>   Interestingly, Denise identified the Midtown CMHT as her preferred team in which to start my research, for a number of particular reasons. First, they are 'having some problems' at the moment. Dealing with social services, she said, is like coming up 'against a brick wall'. She gave me an example. The health side of the team generated a new joint referral form, which was agreed by the ground-level practitioners as appropriate. However, this was not so straightforward with respect to the local authority, who insisted on seeking senior management approval for use of the document. It has now, Denise said, 'disappeared'.
>   (Fieldnotes extract from Health and Social Care, with pseudonyms used for both people and places)

A reflexive approach to data generation in in-depth studies such as Health and Social Care also means maintaining vigilance against the possibility of favouring one respondent's account over another. For example, as a practitioner with a health care rather than a social care background it was important for me not to fall into the trap of assuming that this NHS manager's account of interagency relations was necessarily the 'right' one. Thus, once access had been secured and the process of formal data generation commenced I made the conscious decision to seek out key informants representing all groups and agencies with a stake in service provision in both of my study sites. By adopting a 'neutral' but informed stance in interviews I was able to elicit different, and sometimes competing, accounts of the processes of care organization and delivery.

Once institutional approval for my investigation had been obtained from key individuals located in the NHS trust and social services departments in my study sites it was necessary to negotiate further access to practitioners able and willing to participate in the project. Through them, I needed to negotiate access to service users who might become the starting point for each of my case studies. Possession of practitioner knowledge was important during these processes. My interest was particularly in the examination of occupational and agency interfaces in the context of services provided to people with complex health and social care needs. Recognizing 'complex needs', and thus identifying the kinds of service users to approach to invite their participation in the project, benefited from a practitioner's eye. For example, heavy use of hospital and community mental health services and simultaneous use of care provided by representatives of multiple occupational groups became important considerations during the purposive sampling of case study subjects.

Communicating research ideas to practitioner audiences

In both studies it was necessary to present research ideas, with care, to practitioner audiences. There are different ways in which research ideas can be presented: in writing, through face-to-face meetings, or via intermediaries. In the Stress Study we wanted nurses to complete six separate measures – a considerable request. The questions in these tools touched on sensitive areas. Mailing out batteries of standardized questionnaires of this sort to busy practitioners needs to be done with considerable caution. Without time being taken by researchers to communicate the rationale and aims of a study, or to explain why data are being sought, busy practitioners might reasonably doubt the value of disclosing personal information of this type. Our sole medium for communicating our ideas to individual practitioners in this study was through the letter accompanying each questionnaire pack. Great care therefore had to be taken in the construction of this document. As Figure 8.1 shows, this letter included information signifying the importance of the study for clinical practice, the promise of feedback of the study's findings, and reassurances regarding confidentiality and anonymity.

Most nurses are familiar with the postal or face-to-face survey as a method of data generation. All are likely to have received unsolicited market research questionnaires, or to have been stopped by clipboard-wielding researchers on Saturday afternoons. I knew that few, however, were likely to have participated in in-depth qualitative studies. Many will be unfamiliar with terms like 'ethnography'. In Health and Social Care it was necessary to put into clear and unambiguous language the nature and purpose of my proposed study, and my data generation strategies. In addition, it was important that they were persuaded that the latter were going to produce useful findings. Unlike in the Stress Study two presentation methods were available: the provision of written information, and face-to-face meetings. In face-to-face meetings held in community mental health team (CMHT) premises the reactions of practitioners to my proposals were both interesting and varied. In the CMHT in my first study site (the Midtown team referred to in the fieldnotes extract above) particularly penetrating questions came from a consultant psychiatrist, who wanted to know more about how I intended to manage my dual responsibilities as a researcher and a registered nurse, in the particular context of generating data with vulnerable service users prone to episodes of mental ill-health. Following my presentations some immediately grasped the purpose and methods of my study (the senior mental health social worker in the Midtown CMHT being an excellent example) and worked hard from the outset to facilitate my entry into the field.

Health and Social Care's written practitioner information sheet contained details of the proposed research plan, subtle messages about the importance of the study and, in this case, the credibility of the research team. The information sheet was kept to two sides of A4 paper, but still managed to convey why the study was being proposed, the fact that external funding had been obtained, what taking part in the project would practically mean, and why findings from the study would be of value to the practitioner community. Figure 8.2 reproduces this written information sheet.

Employing practitioner knowledge to develop strategies for data generation

Practice experience helps sharpen research questions and access negotiations with practitioners and service users. In studies like Health and Social Care which employ ethnographic

Figure 8.1 Letter accompanying questionnaire packs used in the All Wales CMHN stress study

[Headed paper]

The all Wales community psychiatric nurses stress study
As part of its ongoing research strategy, the School of Nursing Studies at the University of Wales College of Medicine has been awarded a grant by the General Nursing Council for England and Wales Trust to investigate stress and coping amongst community psychiatric nurses (CPNs) throughout Wales.

Previous research in England, largely completed in the North Thames Regional Health Authority area, has indicated that stress and burnout are significant problems for CPNs and subsequently for their clinical work. It is the intention of the researchers in the first instance to replicate this important original research, using the instruments devised by the North Thames research team.

We have had permission to survey all the CPNs within your Trust. We hope that you will be happy to take the time to fill in the questionnaires in this booklet. A copy of the finished research will be forwarded to your trust at the end of the study.

Your answers to all the questionnaires will remain anonymous and strictly confidential. Please place the completed questionnaire in the envelope provided and return to _____.

There is a possibility due to Trust reconfiguration that you might have completed the questionnaire already. If so then please return the blank questionnaire in the envelope provided.

If you have any queries then please do not hesitate to contact me on [phone number].

Thanking you in advance for your anticipated help.

Please return by / /

Figure 8.2 Information sheet for practitioners developed for the Health and Social Care
           study

[University crest]

Background

How community care is provided to people with severe and enduring mental health
problems is a matter of significance to policy-makers, managers, practitioners and
to individual service users and their carers. The overarching aim in this study is to
examine the ways in which the different agencies and professionals involved in the
provision of care to people with severe mental health problems negotiate their
relative roles and responsibilities. What helps? What hinders? How can community
mental health care be improved? This is an issue of significance and urgency.

Objectives

Objectives for this study include:

- mapping the network of care providers involved in the delivery of services to
  a series of case study subjects over a period of up to four months each;
- locating the findings within the broader policy context at both local and
  national level;
- undertaking detailed study of the ways in which carers manage their respective
  roles and responsibilities in the delivery of health and social services;
- identifying the range of factors related to interagency collaboration which,
  in the opinion of local stakeholders, contribute to or detract from the
  effectiveness and quality of service provision in the study settings;
- feeding back the findings to the study settings, enabling critical reflection on
  the delivery of care and assisting in future service planning;
- using these findings to make recommendations concerning the development
  of roles and responsibilities in the provision of community mental health
  care;
- sharing and disseminating the research findings to a multidisciplinary
  audience.

Research design

Access has been sought to two contrasting study sites within the [name] Health
Authority area. In each site, as full a picture as possible will be sought of the community
care provided to up to four individuals identified as suffering from severe mental
health problems. Established ethnographic case study methods will be employed. In
each case study, the network of care provided will be mapped, in detail, for a period
of up to four months. These networks will be explored using a range of methods:
semi-structured interviews with health and social care providers, informal carers and
clients, and key policy makers and service managers; observation of critical meetings;

continued...

Figure 8.2 continued

and analysis of case notes and key local and national policy documents. Where possible, interviews and observations will be tape-recorded.

Ethical and access considerations

The approval of the [name] Local Research Ethics Committee to undertake this project has been obtained. Potential participants in this study will have the freedom to make an informed decision on whether or not they wish to take part. All participants will, in addition, be assured of their right to withdraw at any point, without this in any way affecting their care and treatment. Pseudonyms will be used for the electronic and paper storage of data. The anonymity of individuals and study sites will be preserved, as far as possible, in the writing up and wider dissemination of findings from the study.

Access to case study subjects will be sought via the hospital and/or community settings. Subjects will be purposively selected. Access will particularly be sought to individuals the complexities of whose needs determine that a wide range of professionals and agencies are involved in their care.

What the study would involve for health, social services and other personnel

In seeking your support for this study I am asking for:

- permission to approach clients who have been identified as experiencing severe and enduring mental health problems to participate in the study;
- permission to observe, and if possible tape record, key events related to the care of the case study subjects (for example, ward rounds, care planning meetings taking place in the community, admission and discharge procedures);
- access to the client/patient records kept by different professionals relating to each case study subject;
- permission to carry out tape-recorded interviews, for approximately one hour each, with the health, social and other workers involved in the provision of care to each case study subject.

Practical benefits

Against the background of complex and shifting health and social policy frameworks, this study will generate new understanding into the ways in which the different professionals and agencies involved in the provision of community mental health care negotiate their respective roles and responsibilities. In particular, insights will be developed into the range of factors which facilitate, and detract from, the delivery of high quality, effective community mental health services. The feeding back of findings to the study sites will enable critical reflection on the delivery of care, and assist in future service planning. Findings will also be used, where appropriate, to make

continued...

Figure 8.2 continued

recommendations concerning the future development of roles and responsibilities in the provision of community mental health care. Finally, this study will generate starting points for further investigations into the delivery of multiagency and multidisciplinary care.

The research team

The principal researcher, Ben Hannigan, has a background in community mental health nursing. Since Autumn 1997 he has worked as a Lecturer in the School of Nursing and Midwifery Studies, UWCM, teaching and researching in the field of community mental health. Research supervision is being provided by Dr Davina Allen and Professor Philip Burnard, both also of the School of Nursing and Midwifery Studies, UWCM. Dr Allen is a skilled ethnographer, whose research interests have focused on changing roles in the health service. She was also a principal researcher on a project funded by the Welsh Office of Research and Development for Health and Social Care which used ethnographic case study methods to investigate the complexities of providing care to people recovering from neurological conditions. Professor Burnard has extensive experience in undertaking and supervising qualitative research, and has written and researched widely in the mental health field.

External support

This study is being supported through the award of a Smith and Nephew Foundation Nursing Research Fellowship.

Further details

For further information, please contact: Ben Hannigan [address and contact details]

methods, it can also help inform the ongoing methodological decision making which takes place during periods of data generation.

Observational methods permit direct access (Burgess, 1984) to the negotiation, provision and receipt of care. This was important in my study, with its focus on the management of roles and responsibilities as these were enacted in everyday workplaces. Self-evidently no researcher can generate observational data on everything taking place in a given social setting (Wolcott, 2001). Researchers therefore have to make (and justify) decisions on what to observe and/or participate in, and practitioner knowledge can assist in this process. As a researcher with community nursing experience I was aware that providers of community care are typically located in dispersed settings, with negotiation of roles and responsibilities often taking place in unpredictable, difficult-to-observe, ways. Practice knowledge led me to a modification of the observational sampling strategy developed in the earlier study from which my design and methods grew in order to encompass the generation of data at events where I knew work-oriented interactions were likely to take place. For example, I made the decision to sample routine multidisciplinary team meetings, at which both business and service user related matters would be discussed. Meetings of this type fulfil various important functions in the weekly rhythms of community teams, such as the receipt and processing of newly referred service users and the discharge of users following completed episodes of care. During my exploration of service user case study subjects' networks of care, practitioner knowledge led me to care planning meetings as an important place for the generation of data relating to the negotiation of interprofessional roles and responsibilities.

Interviews, held with paid health and social care providers, informal carers, service users, policy makers and service managers, assumed an important place in my overall data generation strategy. Knowledge of health and social care professional life and NHS and local authority organizational forms helped my purposive sampling of interview participants able to give me an insight into the general organization of services in my study sites. Practitioner knowledge attuned me to particular lines of enquiry, including systems for the coordination of care across occupational and agency boundaries, eligibility criteria for access to services, and processes for the construction of shared policies.

Completing my data generation strategy was the acquisition and analysis of written records, including local policy documents and practitioners' notes. Like interviews, accessing documents permits investigation into events otherwise inaccessible, or no longer contemporaneous. However, documents come in many different forms, and are produced for different purposes and for different audiences. In health and social care settings practitioner records will often be written with possible future organizational, or even legal, scrutiny in mind. Nurse researchers using written notes as sources of data can use this knowledge in a reflexive manner. In this study, for example, I used notes extensively to help build up a picture of each case study subject's network of care, but did so in the awareness that these often represented a partial, and highly stylized, version of events.

In drawing on their practitioner experiences in ethnographic and other in-depth qualitative investigations, nurse researchers need to exercise care to avoid slipping into previous, perhaps more comfortable, roles. Self-conscious, reflexive, effort may be needed to make the familiar strange and to maintain an analytic edge during data generation (Burgess, 1984). Reed, for example, writes of her first observational experience on a hospital ward for older people in which nothing interesting seemed to happen (Reed, 1995). In fact, complex nursing care had been provided, but as an 'insider' Reed had dismissed this as being too taken-for-granted to be worth recording. Benefiting from possession of an 'outsider's' perspective, Reed's non-nurse research supervisor was able to offer the alternative view of routine nursing care as being both mysterious and worthy of investigation. In a similar way Health and Social Care is also aiming to generate useful new knowledge of the otherwise taken-for-granted provision of everyday services.

Discussion

In this chapter the examples of generating data using standardized measures and using ethnographic methods have illustrated nurse researchers' engagement with different data generation processes and have identified some key learning points.

Ensuring congruence between the study objectives and the data generated

In all studies it is important to achieve congruence between a study's objectives, its theoretical foundations, and the types of data needed and the means of generating these. Achieving this congruence requires decisions to be made, and nurse researchers can creatively draw on their dual practitioner and investigator identities to assist this process. Whereas nurses have sometimes seen the possession of practitioner knowledge as problematic, and as a potential source of bias needing to be overcome (see for a discussion Reed, 1995), we should, perhaps, instead embrace our practitioner experiences as a strength. As the examples in this chapter have shown, practitioner knowledge can help researchers to identify likely sources of data and to assist in the negotiation of access. Practitioner knowledge can also be used to translate research ideas into forms readily understood by practising nurses, and can be drawn on to sensitize researchers to the ways in which invitations to participate in studies are likely to be received by busy clinicians.

The importance of reflexivity

Whilst different strategies place different expectations and demands on nurse researchers, this chapter has also shown that – whatever approach is followed – data generation is always a purposeful activity demanding a reflexive stance. The principle of reflexivity underpins the idea that research always takes place in contexts, shaped to significant degree through an interaction between researcher and researched. The character of data produced in a study is moderated by aspects of the researcher's personal biography and their interaction with research participants. This is a well-established principle in the social sciences. In nursing research, however, reflexive investigators have to give consideration not only to general biographical aspects such as age and gender, but also to their specific occupational backgrounds and practitioner experiences. A self-conscious, reflexive approach includes acknowledgement of the utility and the limitations of practitioner knowledge, and the implications of this for data production.

Conclusion

In both of the case studies used in this chapter 'insider' nursing knowledge was used to inform data generation processes. It is worth reflecting that nurse researchers can be 'insiders' to greater or lesser degrees; for example, in Health and Social Care I carried no ongoing care provision responsibilities for the people who participated as case study subjects. Being an 'insider' has a rather different meaning when, as is described in Chapter 10, practitioners are researching their own clients or educators are researching their own students.

Acknowledgements

The All Wales Community Mental Health Nursing Stress Study research team was led by Professor Philip Burnard, and included Deborah Edwards, Dave Coyle, Anne Fothergill and myself. Health and Social Care for People with Severe Mental Health Problems, a PhD study, is being supervised by Professors Davina Allen and Philip Burnard. I acknowledge their support and guidance here.

References

Abbott, A. (1988) *The System of Professions: An Essay on the Division of Expert Labor*, Chicago, IL: University of Chicago Press.

Allen, D. (2004) 'Ethnomethodological insights into insider-outsider relationships in nursing ethnographies of healthcare settings', *Nursing Inquiry*, 11, 14–24.

Brooker, C. and White, E. (1997) *The Fourth Quinquennial National Community Mental Health Nursing Census of England and Wales*, Manchester and Keele: Universities of Manchester and Keele.

Brown, D., Leary, J., Carson, J., Bartlett, H. and Fagin, L. (1995) 'Stress and the community mental health nurse: the development of a measure', *Journal of Psychiatric and Mental Health Nursing*, 2, 9–12.

Burgess, R.G. (1984) *In the Field: An Introduction to Field Research*, London: Routledge.

Carson, J. and Kuipers, E. (1998) 'Stress management interventions', in S. Handy, J. Carson and B. Thomas (eds) *Occupational Stress: Personal and Professional Approaches*, Cheltenham: Stanley Thornes.

Coffey, A. (1999) *The Ethnographic Self: Fieldwork and the Representation of Identity*, London: Sage.

Edwards, D., Burnard, P., Coyle, D., Fothergill, A. and Hannigan, B. (2000) 'Stress and burnout in community mental health nursing: A review of the literature', *Journal of Psychiatric and Mental Health Nursing*, 7, 7–14.

Ferlie, E. (2001) 'Organisational studies', in N. Fulop, P. Allen, A. Clarke. and N. Black (eds) *Studying the Organisation and Delivery of Health Services: Research Methods*, London: Routledge.

Freidson, E. (1976) 'The division of labour as social interaction', *Social Problems*, 23, 304–13.

Goldberg, D. and Williams, P. (1988) *A Users' Guide to the General Health Questionnaire*, Windsor: NFER-Nelson.

Hammersley, M. and Atkinson, P. (1995) *Ethnography: Principles in Practice*, London: Routledge.

Hughes, E. (1971) *The Sociological Eye: Selected Papers on Work, Self and the Study of Society*, Chicago, IL: Aldine.

Maslach, C., Jackson, S.E. and Leiter, M.P. (1996) *Maslach Burnout Inventory Manual*, Palo Alto, CA: Consulting Psychologists Press.

McElfratick, S., Carson, J., Annett, J., Cooper, C., Holloway, F. and Kuipers, E. (2000) 'Assessing coping skills in mental health nurses: is an occupation specific measure better than a generic coping skills scale?', *Personality and Individual Differences*, 28, 965–76.

Reed, J. (1995) 'Practitioner knowledge in practitioner research', in J. Reed and S. Proctor (eds) *Practitioner Research in Healthcare: The Inside Story*, London: Chapman and Hall.

Rosenberg, M. (1985) *Society and Adolescent Self Image*, Princeton, MA: Princeton University Press.

Wolcott, H.F. (2001) *Writing Up Qualitative Research*, London: Sage.

Wycherley, B. (1987) *The Living Skills Pack*, Bexhill: South East Thames RHA.

Yin, R.K. (1994) *Case Study Research: Design and Methods*, London: Sage.

Chapter 9

Researching practice, service delivery and organization

Lisa Franklin and Chris Martinsen

Introduction

For many nurses, the starting point for their interest in research lies in the workplace. Careers are often launched by an investigation into aspects of their own practice, or the organization in which they work. This presents some very particular challenges, which may only be fully appreciated with hindsight. There is very little literature dealing with this important aspect of nursing research. However, Cormack (2000) identifies ease of access as a benefit of conducting research in a familiar field, and Burnard and Morrison (1994) draw attention to possible constraints, such as the attitudes of key people, which might affect the process. Studies of organizations and their components take many forms, from ethnomethodolgy (see for example Allen, 2004) to cost effectiveness analyses (see for example Thomson, 1999). These do not concern us here, nor does the methodological challenge of conducting research in a familiar field. Rather we will attempt to bring forward some of the less obvious, but equally important issues which we have encountered as insiders studying our own workplace and organization.

This chapter is written by two experienced clinicians who have faced the challenges of this endeavour and lived to tell the story. Lisa Franklin will draw on her experience of studying services for people with or at risk of pressure damage in the organization where she worked. She moved between the worlds of practice and academe to conduct her study. Chris Martinsen remained in his clinical post in Intensive Care. He will recount the successes and frustrations of establishing evidence-based practice systems in that setting.

Case study 1: Researching service organization and delivery: the pressure ulcer problem – Lisa

This work began when I was in full-time clinical practice as a junior sister on a busy vascular unit in a large integrated NHS Trust, where I had been working for eight years. Over this period I had found that patients who suffer with peripheral vascular disease often develop large painful wounds, which can be difficult to manage, and are also often at high risk of pressure ulcer (PU) development. Consequently, I developed considerable clinical expertise and a keen interest in wound care and pressure ulcer management and prevention.

Nationally pressure ulcers continue to occur at a low frequency. The most recent estimate for the UK is that 412,000 individuals develop new pressure damage each year (Bennet et al., 2004). Pressure ulcers have a major impact on the physical, social and financial aspects of patients' lives and are distressing for the people who care for them (National Institute for Clinical Excellence, 2003). The more severe ulcers, grades three and four (European Pressure Ulcer Advisory Panel (EPUAP), 1999) have been seen in clinical practice to require lengthy treatment. This study was initiated by senior personnel in the Health Authority, who were concerned because, although the official view was that severe pressure ulcers had almost disappeared, anecdotal accounts of their continued occurrence regularly surfaced. They therefore proposed a project to clarify the issue and entered into collaboration with the University School of Nursing and the NHS trust in which I was working. This had recently undergone a process of restructuring, bringing acute and community services together into a single organization. The project began in early 2000. A multidisciplinary Project Board was set up, including representatives of the Trust, the University and the Health Authority. It was agreed that the main aim of the study should be:

> To obtain accurate information about the incidence and prevalence of severe pressure ulcers in the community setting served by an acute hospital/community NHS Trust.

Funding was made available to appoint a research associate and the job advertised thus:

> An exciting opportunity exists for a nurse to join a team undertaking a research study to investigate the factors associated with the occurrence of severe pressure ulcers [...] The person appointed will work as a Research Associate conducting fieldwork and will participate in the management of the project as a whole.

I was appointed to this post in early 2001. The Trust agreed to my secondment on a part-time basis, thus I continued to work in my clinical area for two days per week. Until this time my research experience had been limited to the modules studied during my degree, literature reviews for post-registration courses and small-scale project work undertaken as part of my clinical role. With hindsight I have recognized that this was the beginning of a very steep learning curve. I was aware that the work would involve studying my own organization and the working practices of people within it. However, I did not anticipate how difficult this would be.

The methods to be used in the study were discussed by the Project Board. It was agreed that the investigation would employ a variety of methods to address this complex clinical issue and to answer the following research questions:

1   What is the prevalence and incidence of severe (Grade 3 and 4) PU in patients aged 65 and over living in the community (i.e. at home, or in nursing or residential care)?

2   What factors (individual, organizational and service delivery) are associated with the occurrence of severe PU in this population?

3   How can these factors be modified to reduce the risk of deterioration of early PU in this population?

Phase one of the study consisted of: a literature review; a survey of nurses' views about the factors associated with pressure ulcer deterioration at the acute/community interface and collection of epidemiological data from routine and other sources. Phase two consisted of a series of four in-depth case studies, which studied the individual trajectories of individuals who were living at home with pressure damage. The case studies involved observational work, formal and informal interviews with both the patients and their carers, and examination of the patient's general practitioner (GP) and district nursing (DN) records.

The Project Board had agreed that the research associate should be a qualified nurse with relevant clinical experience, because they would bring to the job knowledge of local health care systems, working practices, and direct experience of the research problem. In fact throughout the study I found that my varied clinical experience was indeed extremely valuable in the project's development and conduct and helped to provide a sensitive and insightful approach to this piece of work. Having insider knowledge of the organization meant that I had few problems in obtaining initial support for the study and permission to access staff. For example, in my nursing role I already had developed a close working relationship with the Trust's specialist nurses in wound healing and hence gained a lot of support from them during the study. A second advantage of being an experienced clinician within the organization was that I had already formulated certain ideas, which could only have been produced through experience of that organization. However, I recognized that these ideas could potentially impact upon the study and lead to researcher bias. Bias has been described as a tendency to produce and interpret data in a way which leans towards conclusions which match the researcher's own inclinations (Hammersley and Gomm, 1997).

Mindful of this I documented a series of foreunderstandings (Ashworth, 1987) to describe the beliefs that I had that related to the research at the start of the study and prior to commencing phase two. This was one way of achieving the reflexive approach to data generation which has been described in Chapter 8. I was very aware of these during the data collection processes and revised them at the end of the study. For example, at the start of the study I believed that communication between community staff and ward staff is often inadequate (on admission to hospital as well as on discharge). Consequently communication between the acute and community settings was purposively included in the interview schedule in phase one of the study. Care was taken to ensure that both positive and negative views on communication could be expressed and I looked carefully for counter-examples. The interviews confirmed that, although some good practice exists, community nurses are often dissatisfied with the information that they receive before visiting the patient, the transfer letter limits the information given, and hospital nurses do not seem to know how their community colleagues operate. The hospital nurses reported fewer problems with communication, but suggested it would be helpful if DN records were sent in with the patient to hospital. These findings enabled us to suggest ways of improving communication between the two settings.

Hence, I found that although my beliefs naturally impacted upon the study they helped enormously in the planning of both phases. I believe that if a researcher with no nursing knowledge had carried out the project certain key issues may not have been addressed. However, a person from outside the organization would have suffered fewer of the conflicts to be described in the following section. These might be considered as disadvantages of being an insider, although it could be argued that their creative resolution is a positive feature.

Throughout the project I found the experience of managing a dual role within the organization very intense and experienced some degree of role conflict. This took a number of forms including: full-time/part-time worker conflict when seconded from my clinical post; insider/outsider conflict when moving between practice and academia; nurse/researcher conflict when observing practice and even acute/community conflict when moving between the two sectors of the newly integrated Trust.

On a very practical level, becoming a part-timer in my clinical work introduced a conflict around the time I could spend there. This pitfall had been anticipated at an early stage and I had undertaken preparatory work looking at effective organizational and workload management skills. However, as the project progressed the demands of the research meant that this could easily have been a full-time job on its own. I was increasingly aware of the workload pressures on colleagues in my clinical area, during a time of transition in the NHS as a whole, and I still felt a strong pull from that direction. This became an extremely demanding period. To help to deal with this I employed reflective skills and sought the support of experienced colleagues in both the clinical area and the research setting.

As a practising nurse I had spent many years in a highly pressured and stressful clinical environment. I was very well aware that involvement in research can be viewed as extra work for health care professionals who are already dealing with their own heavy workloads. Because of this, the project was designed to disrupt working practices as little as possible, but conflict still occurred. I first experienced this during phase one of the study when I found that the nursing staff whom I wished to interview were already working under tremendous pressures. I felt very uneasy about this, remembering only too well the annoyance that I had felt in the past when approached by researchers during my clinical work: My response at that time had been 'why couldn't they see how much work I had to do already!' As an organizational insider, I was automatically giving the needs of the service priority over the demands of the research project.

I also felt some conflict of loyalties when recruiting. Hampton, et al. (1998) described a similar situation, whereby their access to potential research participants was limited during their study of pressure ulcer development in the community. They experienced frustrations and difficulties when liaising with district nurses and carers in order to gain access to potential participants. In this way, nurses and carers were 'gate-keeping'. I also experienced these frustrations. However, if a district nurse said that it was not appropriate to approach a patient I would try to discuss this with them but ultimately had to trust their judgement, as they were acting as the patient's advocate.

Contacting the DNs was difficult in itself, as they were frequently out of the office. I felt it was not appropriate to contact them on their mobile phones as they would either be driving or giving direct patient care. So I often found myself leaving numerous unanswered messages on clinic answer phones. I felt my loyalties lay with ensuring that I impacted as little as possible on the nursing workloads. At the same time, I was conscious of the need to meet the objectives of the Project Board team in recruiting subjects to the study. This created considerable stress as I tried to deal with these conflicting pressures.

During the course of the study I was based in an office in the School of Nursing and Midwifery Studies Research Centre where I worked alongside a group of researchers of varying levels of experience. However, whilst I was very much an insider in the clinical setting, I found that this was a very different environment in which I was, although welcome, effectively an outsider. I was interested to observe the contrast between the way that the researchers and clinicians thought about and carried out their work. The researchers had less idea about the reality of current nursing practice and for them the research is naturally their priority. Clinicians, however, seem to have research much lower down in their priorities as they battle against ever-increasing workloads. Researchers also work in a much less structured environment. I was used to the hierarchy of the nursing team and having a lot of my work time planned for me. For example someone else decided my shift patterns. When I moved to this small team of researchers I found myself managing my own time, and at times I felt very vulnerable. In addition, researchers do not have policies and procedures in place to govern their practice as clinical nurses do, and are obliged to think for themselves much more. For example, if during my nursing practice I needed to set up a pump which would deliver a controlled drug there would be a protocol in place to guide me throughout every step of the process. However, when I wanted to carry out semi-structured interviews there were no organizational guidelines in place to help me to do this. Although there are obvious controls in place within the research setting, such as research governance, these are less prescriptive than in the service setting. As clinicians we often have to utilize both our clinical judgement and effective problem-solving skills when working day-to-day. However, our thinking is much more applied and takes place within a framework for safe practice. Researchers appear to easily apply their thinking processes to a set of data and bring their own ideas and thoughts.

It took a long time for me to learn to think in the much more open manner that researchers do and also to value more my own thoughts and opinions.

I found it difficult to make the transition from clinician to researcher and come to terms with my role. I went from being an experienced nurse working in a structured environment with clear-cut practice guidelines to follow, to a novice researcher who felt completely lost as I tried to find my way. As the study proceeded, I moved regularly between the two worlds of practice and academe. Each of the phases of the study provided me with the opportunity to learn new skills, not just research techniques. On reflection, this experience of working in a different environment helped me to become more detached from my own organization and to see it through fresh eyes.

The final phase of the study involved case studies. The objective here was to conduct an in-depth examination of a small number of cases of people with established severe ulcers, to identify the organizational and other factors associated with their onset. An element of each case study was observational work, for which I had negotiated the permission of the patients and their nurses. As a nurse I soon realized that observational opportunities were going to be limited, as the patient's privacy and dignity would need to be maintained in their home. However, with the permission of the patients and their nurses, I was able to observe at least one wound dressing change for each patient. Here I experienced the care giver/researcher conflict. I was frequently a frustrated nurse as I was unable to contribute to the care and had to step back and observe. In an attempt to address this I completed my field notes in two sections – what I thought as a nurse and what I thought as a researcher. This helped me to separate out my thoughts and to retain distance, whilst still allowing me to document my nursing thoughts.

Although the pre-study information had emphasized that I would not be looking at individual nursing practice it was inevitable that some of the nurses involved would feel that this was happening. Consequently, the observational situations had to be handled sensitively, especially as, after integration of acute and community services, the respondents were working for the same organization as myself. I wore a uniform, for the benefit of the patient, and assisted with the care provision when appropriate, for example helping to move the patient or make them comfortable under the direction of the care-giving nurse. This seemed to help both nurse and patient feel more at ease. I had anticipated that I might observe inappropriate care and had formulated an action plan to deal with this eventuality. Only once did I feel some genuine concern about the care that was being provided for the pressure ulcer. On this occasion the situation was reported to the Specialist Nurse in Wound Healing and was addressed effectively. Since the possibility that the patients involved would be discussed with the Specialist Nurse had been made clear in the pre-study information, it was possible to do this openly. The potentially damaging interpretation that this was covert surveillance of community nursing practice was thus avoided.

This first case study illustrates the uphill and sometimes bewildering path that I took as a novice researcher conducting research in my own organization. A number of benefits and drawbacks of the insider position have been identified. In recent years, the governance of research has been strengthened (Department of Health, 2005; Wales Office of Research and Development for Health and Social Care, 2001). The researcher practitioner relationship has come under scrutiny, in recognition of the conflicts occurring when researcher and caregiver are one and the same. The emphasis has been on the establishment of systems to avoid the bias that may be introduced to clinical trials if the researchers are also the carers of participants (see Chapter 10). Much less attention has been paid to the other conflicts such as those I experienced when conducting research in my own organization.

Case study 2: Researching practice: a sticky experience – Chris

Some years ago as a senior clinical nurse in a large and expanding Intensive Care Unit (ICU) I was more committed than most to the concept of evidence-based practice. This included a desire to carry out primary research, but as I wished to continue caring for patients and felt that generating evidence should be an intrinsic part of the clinical nursing role, I was not tempted to apply for 'traditional' research nurse posts.

My dream of primary research was turned into reality when I was contacted by a former colleague who now worked for a commercial clinical trials company. They had been asked, by a manufacturer, to identify a suitable centre to carry out a study for which they had already developed the research protocol. My former colleague immediately thought of our Intensive Care Unit as a potentially suitable setting and, knowing my interest in research, came to me as a first contact. I was inclined to jump at this opportunity, which, having come my way by such a fortunate series of circumstances, seemed to be the work of the hand of destiny. The study was a small randomized controlled trial comparing the cost effectiveness of two transparent dressings for use on peripheral intravenous catheters: hence the title of this case study. (I soon discovered that a sense of humour is an essential attribute of the field researcher.)

After a series of meetings the Clinical Director approved the undertaking of the research and the protocol was deemed practicable in the clinical environment. I was appointed Principal Investigator. This involved first preparatory work; organizing and delivering the educational sessions for staff and recruiting and training the members of the monitoring group. In addition, I had to ensure the efficient progress of the study. This included: making sure that all necessary materials required to carry out the study were available; making up recruitment packs; ensuring that recruitment was in accordance with the randomization procedure; being responsible for data collection and ensuring that procedures were carried out according to protocol. The study was to be in full compliance with the 'ICH guideline for good clinical practice' for conduct of research (International Committee on Harmonisation and Good Clinical Practice, 1996). A clinical trials company was therefore appointed to externally monitor the data collection and data analysis. I was responsible for facilitating the external monitoring process and attending to any queries. I was given five working days of dedicated time for this process, most of which was taken up in the preparations. Some of the work was done in my clinical time as opportunity and circumstance allowed and inevitably I carried out a good deal of work in 'my own time'. (I had realized from the outset that this would be the case.)

The costs of materials including, the production of Case Report Forms (CRFs), external monitoring of the study and data analysis were to be borne by the sponsor. A small per capita fee was to be paid to the Directorate for each completed CRF. This would not be sufficient to employ external researchers, but in any case the nature of the study suggested that most of the ICU nursing workforce would need to be involved in the collection of data. This was because the recruitment of subjects would be not only opportunistic but also in a short time frame. (If a patient needs peripheral intravenous access they usually need it immediately.) The sponsoring company was prepared to fund the education and training of staff members in the use of the research protocol and data collection.

This approach was expected to be practicable as both the protocol and CRF were relatively simple and the data to be collected consisted mainly of routine observations made as part of the normal care of the patient receiving peripheral intravenous therapy (e.g. position of catheter insertion and condition of the dressing). The only additional work required was, therefore, completion of the CRF, a process which would take about five minutes (provided the individual felt confident in the process). This was not therefore expected to be a great burden to place on the staff. Yet to my surprise, many of my colleagues found the task of filling out the CRF daunting. I had not expected this, since these practitioners are used to meticulous observation, complex record keeping and making critical decisions associated with potentially very serious consequences. Despite this, they often appeared to need reassurance that they had filled in the CRF correctly (even though they usually had done so) and found it difficult to believe that the task was as straightforward as it seemed. I wondered why they needed so much support and reassurance to carry out what I assumed to be a relatively simple process. In retrospect I think that this may have been, in part, a consequence of the educational sessions which we gave to prepare colleagues for their role in which, due to our lack of experience, we may have reinforced rather than removed some of the mystique surrounding research.

I had anticipated that nurses would be as keen as I to take part in the study. The outcome of the study would be the identification of the most effective dressing and this had the potential to reduce some of the risks associated with the administration of intravenous therapy (e.g. phlebitis, extravasations, infection) and to save nursing time in reducing the frequency of changing dressings. In other words, I had assumed that colleagues would share my view that the project was 'a good thing'.

I also expected that use of the research protocol and the stringency of observation and data collection would in itself improve the quality of associated care (this was confirmed by clinical audit). Further, I anticipated that nurses would be more willing to take part because the study was nurse led and its benefits were of direct relevance to nursing practice. This, I thought would overcome the antipathy of nurses to collecting data for projects (e.g. medical research) in which they have no other involvement or interest. These expectations all arose from my insider role within the unit. Unlike Lisa, I did not go through the process of articulating these prior beliefs.

I was also aware of some of the potential problems that might arise in collecting data of the kind required. Since so many individuals were to be involved, and the pace of work in ICU can be so intense, problems of accuracy and inter-rater variability were anticipated. Therefore, in addition to the external monitoring, a small group of nurses was recruited to perform close internal monitoring of the study aiming to check adherence to the protocol, observations and the CRFs on, at least, a daily basis. Their function was also to help and advise other nurses in recruiting patients into the study, following the protocol and completing the CRFs.

We were fortunate in that for most of the period of data collection there was no shortage of potential recruits. Indeed clinical workload sometimes prevented our ability to recruit. We only had a few refusals of consent to participate, and had an acceptably low level of failure to complete data collection, most of which was due to changes in the recruit's circumstances rather than protocol violation.

In the event, it proved much harder than expected to secure commitment from all colleagues. Several reasons for this suggest themselves. First and foremost was the relative priority accorded to research and practice; as when attending to the critically ill, nurses clearly have to give priority to the necessary minute to minute interventions. Second, it proved impracticable to arrange the duty roster so that either a group member or myself was always on duty. Finally, monitoring group members, who had their own clinical workload, could not always find the time for monitoring and advisory activities. Calls for help, in many cases just for reassurance, as previously suggested, were frequent. This difficulty was exacerbated by the fact that they encountered a degree of resentment from some colleagues who felt they had to take over some of the monitors' 'normal workload'.

Despite these problems the project was completed, within the agreed period of time, to the size of study initially agreed. At this point, as hoped and surmised, a statistically significant result was achieved. This demonstrated that the one dressing was, by specified criteria, both more cost effective and clinically effective than the other. This result was of clinical importance and was used to improve local standards of care, contributing to the profile of the unit as a centre of excellence. The sponsoring manufacturers deemed the results sufficient for their purpose and have quoted the study as support for the product in marketing literature. The findings of the project and subsequent audit work gave rise to four presentations at national and international gatherings (Martinsen, 1998, 1998a, 1998b, 2000) where I had the opportunity to discuss my work. These conferences were not only great from the educational and travel point of view but also offered networking opportunities, including meeting some revered names from the literature, spawning further ideas and aspirations on my part. I felt regret that the many colleagues who had contributed to the work were unable to share this experience and hoped that some would perhaps follow my example in taking opportunities to engage in research and enjoy the benefits.

My first piece of clinically focused research in the critical care setting led me to question the place of research in the clinical nurse's role and in the organization. In the one-to-one nursing situation that was the setting for this study, the individual nurse is very focused on 'their patient'. There are times when the nurse has to be absent for a period, for example, to take a break, fetch equipment or help a colleague and neighbouring nurses will readily care for the patient under those circumstances. This is an accepted part of the unit culture. However, the monitoring group encountered a different attitude when they took breaks to carry out research related activities. There was some resentment that they were leaving 'their' patients in the care of others to perform what were seen as administrative rather than clinically relevant duties. Why should this be?

Certainly over recent years nurses have been prepared for their role by higher education and the emphasis on evidence-based practice would suggest that research should be fundamentally incorporated in nursing culture. But, as we have seen in Part 1, the appropriate level of research engagement in clinical roles has not been clearly defined. This has an impact on the commitment of nurses and makes the task of conducting research in one's own organization even more difficult. On the other hand, the organizational aims of most NHS trusts include a commitment to research and evidence-based practice. Senior nurses have been appointed to develop and implement nursing research strategies. My study was clearly seen as having some value by my Trust. Managers of my directorate have used this activity in recruitment processes, by displaying the conference posters at job fairs in the UK and abroad. But in practice it has proved very difficult to secure support to take undertake further developments in evidence-based care. This causes a frustration which I am sure is shared by many colleagues. It seems as if the organizational view is 'no you can't implement this change without evidence' but 'no I can't provide you with resource to find or generate this evidence'!

Discussion

These two case studies have illustrated how we, as two experienced clinical nurses with enquiring minds, began to engage in research as novice research producers whilst remaining grounded in clinical practice within our own organizations. We have identified the advantages of our insider status in terms of knowledge of the organization and personal relationships. In both cases, the impetus for the study was external, but provided the rare opportunity for which we had been waiting. This reflects the difficulty of securing resources to allow clinicians to instigate and carry out research on their own practice.

Finding an insider-voice

The two projects were initiated by external stakeholders rather than ourselves. They had representatives who had no practical experience of the clinical environment in which the data was to be collected, and the research protocols were generated in this situation. We both felt at times that their expectations of the practicality of data collection were unrealistic, and this often led to self-doubt and fears about our competency. However, we were both fortunate to have people amongst the stakeholders who did have direct experience of our workplaces who were able to allay our fears. We therefore consider that it is important for nurses researching their own practice or organization to make proper use of their insider status by ensuring that their voices are truly heard during project planning and that their experience of the practicalities of the situation is fully utilized.

There is, of course, a dilemma for the nurse who wishes to capitalize on one of the few opportunities that come their way. How assertive should they be in pointing up practical difficulties if they wish to secure the job or contract? Having obtained the opportunity, should they then point out problems of which they were previously aware? How will it look if, having taken on the project, they cannot deliver because of problems that might have been foreseen? These questions show the need for skills that are rarely discussed and certainly were not included in our repertoires at the time. We recommend that these receive more attention in the education of nurse research producers.

Standing in the shoes of significant others

Our experiences contrasted in that Lisa needed to examine current practice, at individual and organizational level whereas Chris was concerned with a comparison of two interventions. Consequently, Lisa spent considerable time examining her prior assumptions about the project, whereas Chris assumed all right thinking people would see the project as a good thing. Both of us underestimated the extent to which the project would be affected by the attitudes of colleagues and, even more so, our own beliefs about those attitudes. In each of our situations we had an awareness of how things were done and talked about in a particular part of the organization at that particular time, what might be called the organizational discourse. This was both an advantage and a disadvantage.

Our experiences have led us to identify useful strategies for conducting research of this nature. In the first place, in order to secure commitment from colleagues, it is essential that the question to be addressed is one that most feel is worth making an effort to answer. The true demands of participation need to be weighed against the benefits that people who work in the organization believe to be likely. A full exploration of both demands and beliefs is essential during the planning stage, followed by modification of the project and further negotiation, if necessary, to take account of these realities. (This demonstrates the importance of the influencer role which has been discussed in Chapter 5.)

Participants need to have a sense of ownership and be given credit for their work. This might be recorded in their personal professional development plan and curriculum vitae. Feedback of results can be used to demonstrate consequential improved local standards of care. Publication of results is likely to generate pride in the department or unit as a centre of excellence, but care is needed to ensure that all contributions are properly acknowledged; otherwise some resentment may cloud future relationships.

Securing institutional support

As nurses we were insiders to the professional culture and subject to the professional discourse described in Part 1, in which, when the chips are down, clinical practice has priority over all other activities. Chris was surprised to find that research activities were resented when they appeared to intrude on clinical time. Lisa, from her prior experience, recalled the impact of research on her clinical work. We both worked very hard, maybe too hard, to ensure that the research did not impact upon clinical practice. Perhaps if we had not been so aware of the demands of practice and the adverse view of anything that got in its way, we might have been less concerned about this and encountered less role conflict. In retrospect, we can see that we were assuming all the responsibility for protecting practice from the demands of research. In our view, researchers in this position need to have the necessary support to give the demands of their research full attention. If this type of research is to succeed it is essential that senior managers are fully engaged in research of this type. Both the researcher and their colleagues must receive support in the form of both time out from their clinical role and the provision of the necessary resources if researcher role conflict is to be reduced.

Conclusion

We have found working as an organizational insider to be subject to multiple influences that need to be brought into the open. The scarcity of opportunities often makes it necessary for aspiring researchers to accept projects that are on offer, which are shaped by the initiating stakeholders' agenda. Professional, managerial and organizational discourses influence the attitude of colleagues, their commitment to the project and their relationships, present and future, with the researcher. Insider knowledge brings many advantages but also lays the researcher open to a variety of role ambiguities and conflicts. The research producer in this situation requires not only competence in the particular research field but also the appropriate support mechanisms and a range of other skills which have been suggested in this chapter. Clarifying and defining these skills for the purposes of role descriptions will help to ensure that these valuable opportunities yield their full value to all concerned.

Acknowledgements

Lisa Franklin's study was supported by a grant from the Wales Office of Research and Development for Health and Social Care. Thanks are due also to Professor P.A. Lyne and Professor D.A. Allen of the Nursing Health and Social Care Research Centre, School of Nursing and Midwifery Studies Cardiff University, for the considerable support that they provided for this study. Chris Martinsen's study was sponsored by the 3M Company. Thanks to all colleagues who participated in the data collection.

References

Allen, D. (2004) 'Ethnomethodological insights into insider-outsider relationships in nursing ethnographies of healthcare settings', *Nursing Inquiry,* 11, 14–24.
Ashworth, P. (1987) *Adequacy of Description: The Validity of Qualitative Findings in Education Management*, Sheffield: Sheffield City Polytechnic, Department of Education Management.
Bennet, G., Dealey, C. and Posnett, J. (2004) 'The cost of pressure ulcers in the UK', *Age and Aging*, 33, 230–5.

Burnard, P. and Morrison, P. (1994) *Nursing Research in Action: Developing Basic Skills*, Basingstoke: Macmillan.

Cormack, D.F.S. (2000) *The Research Process in Nursing*, Oxford: Blackwell Science.

Department of Health (2005) *Research Governance Framework for Health and Social Care*, London: Department of Health.

European Pressure Ulcer Advisory Panel (EPUAP) (1999) *Pressure Ulcer Prevention Guidelines*, Oxford: EPUAP.

Hammersley, M. and Gomm, R. (1997) 'Bias in social research', *Sociological Research Online*, 2.

Hampton, J., Higgins, J. and Cronin, V. (1998) 'Research involving housebound people', *Journal of Community Nursing*, 12, 36–7.

International Committee on Harmonisation and Good Clinical Practice (1996) *Guideline for Good Practice* (ICH Harmonised Tripartite Guideline).

Martinsen, C. (1998) 'A randomised study to assess dressing performance of two peripheral intravenous cannula dressings', Welsh Intensive Care Society Conference, Portmeirion.

Martinsen, C., Findlay, G.P. and Smithies, M.N. (1998a) 'A randomised study to assess dressing performance of two peripheral intravenous cannula dressings', European Society of Intensive Care Medicine 11th Annual Conference, Stockholm, Sweden.

—— (1998b) 'A randomised study to assess dressing performance of two peripheral intravenous cannula dressings', Annual Conference of the British Association of Critical Care Nurses, Manchester.

Martinsen, C., Hughes, A. and Smithies, M.N. (2000) 'Baseline audit of manipulation and management of intravenous delivery systems', 20th International Symposium on Intensive Care and Emergency Medicine, Brussels, Belgium.

National Institute for Clinical Excellence (2003) *Pressure Ulcer Risk Assessment and Prevention, Including the use of Pressure Relieving Equipment (Beds, Mattresses and Overlays) for the Prevention of Pressure Ulcers in Primary and Secondary Care*, London: National Institute for Clinical Effectiveness.

Thomson, J.S. (1999) 'The economics of preventing and treating pressure ulcers: a pilot study', *Journal of Wound Care*, 8, 312–16.

Wales Office of Research and Development for Health and Social Care (2001) *Research Governance Framework for Health and Social Care in Wales*, Cardiff: Wales Office of Research and Development for Health and Social Care.

Chapter 10

Researching your own clients/students

Lesley Lowes and Keith Weeks

Introduction

This chapter deals with the sometimes contentious issue of nurses conducting research involving people to whom they provide professional services. The relationships between nurses and their clients is of a particular kind and, as we have seen in Chapter 2, that between nurse educator and student tends to be more sustained than is the case in many disciplines. Therefore conducting research in which clients or students are *directly* involved as participants takes place at the sensitive interface with professional practice and requires attention to the professional and political issues existing here. It is often the case that a research project will *indirectly* involve the researcher's clients or students, for example through the use of their records, their work or by evaluation of their practice. The implications of doing this are seldom considered, but, as we will show, they too require attention if the work is to be done in such a way that the autonomy of the research subjects is to be respected.

Researchers within the naturalistic paradigm work closely with research participants and the complex relationships between researcher, participant and data generation have been widely debated. Studies involving clients or students are a special case of this kind of work and many nurse researchers adopt this stance, since it reflects their professional caring ethos. For biomedical scientists, however, the basis of experimental research is that the field should be uncontaminated and therefore any relationship between the researcher and subjects outside the research setting is anathema, since it is seen as a source of uncontrolled variation. Nursing research takes place in an arena where conflicts between these two positions often occur and the disagreements about questions of using clients as research subjects provide an exemplar case of the interaction between these powerful forces.

Both authors of this chapter have undertaken research involving clients or students with whom they also have a professional role. Lesley Lowes will show how she worked directly with families to whom she delivered care. Keith Weeks will describe a complex project in which students were directly and indirectly involved at different times and in different ways.

Case study 1: Researching your own clients – Lesley

Many nursing research projects originate from researchers' professional concerns. For example, Long (1997) investigated the needs of parents of newborn infants hospitalized for gastro-intestinal surgery on her ward, and Campbell (1999), a lecturer in oncology nursing, explored the feelings of oncology patients nursed in protective isolation. This was true in my case when, in 1996, I was working as a G grade paediatric diabetes specialist nurse, with home management of newly diagnosed children a large part of my role. I became increasingly concerned about the demands placed on parents at this difficult time in their lives and decided that a study of their experiences would be valuable both to the service and my own development. For my doctoral thesis therefore, I decided to undertake a longitudinal qualitative project that explored parents' experience of having a child diagnosed with diabetes and managed at home (Lowes, 2000; Lowes et al., 2004).

Participants had to be parents of children with newly diagnosed diabetes who were clinically well at presentation and managed at home. (Full details of the study are in Lowes, 2000; Lowes et al., 2004; Lowes et al., 2005). Working with my own clients was a matter of necessity, since the only other centres practising home management at that time were geographically distant, so there was no possibility of conducting the study on another site. Therefore, the only available population was one for which I was also one of the paediatric diabetes specialist nurses providing clinical care. My medical consultant colleague, an experienced quantitative researcher, was closely involved with the study but freely admitted that he had little knowledge of the qualitative process. He was, however, open to new ideas and took the trouble to develop an understanding of them. Nevertheless, I was conscious of his concerns relating to contact with research subjects and was at pains to ensure that my case for working in this way was as rigorous as possible.

Although I was very clear about the broad area of study from the outset, I still experienced some of the dilemmas described by Edmunds in Chapter 6 of this book in refining the focus and satisfying a range of conditions and expectations. I first became aware that this work might be viewed as an *evaluation* of home management when the Local Research Ethics Committee raised concerns about the introduction of bias through parents appraising the service when the researcher was also their main caregiver. To address their concern, I agreed that other diabetes nurses would look after 50 per cent of the sample. Subsequent data analysis showed no difference in findings between the two groups of parents but the distinction between the groups was inevitably blurred because in reality I had unavoidable contact with all the parents during clinic visits or via the on-call telephone.

The qualitative research literature emphasizes that researchers' backgrounds, prior knowledge and preconceptions of the study phenomenon are interconnected with the research, influencing their responses to participants, data generation and analysis (Rodgers and Cowles, 1993). Qualitative interviewers develop consciousness of what they bring to the interaction (Streubert, 1995). I acknowledged that I approached this work with much previous engagement with the study phenomenon. For example, I understood the practical details of the management of this chronic condition very well and knew what parents who managed their children at home from diagnosis would have to do. I appreciated the long-term, life-threatening consequences of poor glycaemic control and had previously accompanied parents as they came to realize what the future might hold and faced the challenge of keeping their child safe. I had had intensive clinical contact with parents in the population available for study and had seen something of their emotional response to the diagnosis. As a specialist nurse, I had formed my own view of the demands made by home management and I also brought life experiences, including those as mother of three children, to the enterprise. It was clear to me that my prior experience would form an important part of the context for data generation but, before I reached that stage, I found that it had an impact on the question of recruiting participants and particularly, of securing their consent.

Obtaining consent

It was my intention to begin the longitudinal study with each family as early as possible and so I needed to ask parents if they would be willing to participate two days after they had received the diagnosis that their child had diabetes. I was concerned about introducing this request at such a time, as I had observed many parents becoming upset after their child's diagnosis and believed that I too would have been distressed under these circumstances. I anticipated that a request to participate in research, particularly if it involved a difficult choice, would be an extra stressor. For many of the families, I would also be a pivotal member of the team providing care. My dilemma was how to manage this complex relationship and ensure that parents were able to give informed consent when they were dependent on my support in so many ways. Were they able to make rational and informed decisions about whether or not to consent at such a distressing and difficult time? Would they actually feel free to refuse, or would they be reluctant to withhold consent for fear of upsetting me, either through a sense of obligation or the prospect of reciprocal benefit? (Van Stuijvenberg et al., 1998). As I thought through all these issues, my motivation for undertaking the study was questioned by others and myself. Was I merely attempting to reassure myself that home management, to which our service was committed, was appropriate for parents? If it were not, would the study come to this conclusion and what would be the consequences if it did?

Such questions forced me back, time and time again, to regain clarity about what was actually being attempted. I had to be very clear that the purpose was to explore parents' experience, and not to evaluate service provision. I had to remind myself that, as a carer, it was appropriate for me to ask about their experiences, so the topic had legitimacy within the client-professional relationship, as well as being the subject of the research. On reflection, I concluded that, if they were given all the relevant information, parents had the autonomy and the right to decide whether or not to participate. Having worked through all these questions I felt sufficiently prepared and confident to begin recruiting. I was at pains to ensure that parents understood the purpose of the study and that they were free to withdraw at any time. Somewhat to my surprise, every one of the 38 parents who met the study criteria agreed to participate and none subsequently dropped out. This increased my concerns and prompted me to explore their motivation to consent at the end of the study. Most parents described reasons related to altruism but one father said:

> I thought, why the bloody hell is she coming in at this stage of it, you know. Can't you leave us in peace for a while? And that was my honest reaction. We thought, oh, do we really want to do this?

Subsequently all the parents described the opportunity to talk about their experiences as helpful, a finding that I found reassuring, though ultimately it is impossible to determine whether, or to what extent, my dual role influenced parents' decisions to participate and persist.

Data generation

The planned method of data generation was the interview and I was very aware of the methodological debates concerning interview-based studies. It was important that my findings should be sufficiently trustworthy to inform service provision. My thinking was influenced by the work of Ashworth (1987), who believes demonstrable validity is possible in qualitative research. I developed an 'audit trail', in which clear documentation of the research methods, contextual data, my self-awareness and choices made during analysis and interpretation allowed readers to follow or 'audit' my thinking and reasoning, and to scrutinize for bias or error (Koch, 1996; Guba, 1981; Rodgers and Cowles, 1993). Later, I explored the data in different ways, challenging its interpretation through critical reflection and testing preconceptions and hypotheses. For example, the data generated by the interviews did not support my preconception about home management being too demanding for all parents and, thus, quite early on in the research, I rejected this assumption. The above processes are relevant to all interview-based studies, but in my case it was necessary to deal with an unusual researcher–participant relationship, in which power issues between the researcher and the researched were of particular concern.

Any interview, even an unstructured one, is always guided by the interviewer to some degree. Bowler (1997) points out that the very fact that the researcher is collecting data about participants places the latter in a subordinate position. When this interaction takes place in the context of a client-professional relationship, as I discovered, the dilemma is brought into even sharper focus. I was very aware that, in inviting parents to participate, I could inadvertently be making use of unacknowledged power differentials. If I was seen as more powerful, parents' responses could have been inhibited and they may have disclosed only what they thought I wanted to hear.

To deal with these concerns, I reiterated the purpose of the study to parents before each interview, emphasizing that I was interested in *their* accounts of the way that they had coped with home management of their child's diabetes. I looked for evidence that parents' accounts were designed to please, present themselves in a favourable light or manipulate the situation. In practice, I found that parents were rarely hesitant in discussing the topic. Some expressed the view that they could comfortably talk about such times knowing that I was aware of the anxieties and difficulties they had experienced. Their accounts were not always positive, and they frequently talked about when they felt they had not coped or had made mistakes. In addition, they mentioned events that did not meet their expectation of the service:

> The [doctor] we saw [in clinic] … she was horrible, wasn't she? She said to me 'Oh, you obviously haven't come to terms with it, have you?' You know, about the diabetes and everything. And I said 'No, I suppose I haven't, have I?' I felt like walking out because her attitude was terrible.

Parents rarely mentioned my clinical involvement in their care or sought clinical advice during an interview. As far as I was able to discern, with one exception, no parent made any attempt to secure additional care or resources for themselves or their child. In the one case (see below) additional support was secured for a family with particular needs. These observations led me to conclude that any perceived imbalance of power had minimal effect on the trustworthiness of the data, when presented to the reader in the context of the audit trail.

As the findings from my study emerged, I was surprised by the intensity of the experiences reported by parents. The diagnosis was described as a sudden and devastating experience, eliciting feelings of loss, shock, sadness and distress. Recounting this experience, several parents, particularly mothers, became upset, which raised a concern regarding non-maleficence. The duty of not inflicting harm is an important consideration in any research (Lyon and Walker, 1997), and the possibility of parents becoming distressed was considered in depth before my study commenced. As a researcher, I was aware that interviewing, is likely to stimulate many emotions and may lead to self-reflection, catharsis and considerable self-disclosure by participants (May, 1991). Since I was also a carer, my dual role caused additional concerns, and sometimes affected the way I interacted with parents. For example, I knew that one mother had suffered a severe bout of depression about 18 months before her daughter was diagnosed. This made me reluctant to pursue emotional issues unless the mother brought them up herself, because I was unsure as to whether asking the mother to confront her feelings could be harmful to her well being. Thus, my prior knowledge of the study participants, derived from my clinical role, acted as a constraint in the interview situation.

My ability to influence the caring processes for the families gave rise to a further dilemma in the case of the parents of a 12-year-old boy, as shown in this field note extract:

> It was revealed that (son) is hitting his mother and sister (enough to cause nasty bruising). I find this disturbing … it is difficult in this situation to divorce my clinical role from my research role. This has implications for child protection … these parents have asked for help throughout the interview. They have obviously sought outside help to no avail, and I will be unable to ignore this after the interview. They need help and, ethically, I cannot ignore this.

These parents requested psychiatric or psychological intervention for their son. I could not morally, professionally or ethically, ignore their request. Consequently, I arranged counselling sessions for this family before their third interview. It could be suggested that therapeutic intervention before completion of all the interviews could alter the outcomes of interviews conducted after the therapy. This would raise the ethical issue of the needs of participants versus successful completion of the research. As May (1991) concludes, though, individual researchers must handle these situations according to their previous experience, skill level and judgement, based on the surrounding circumstances. I believed that, because the psychological intervention for this family would have occurred whether or not they had taken part in the study, my actions should not be construed as introducing a bias.

The emotions of the researcher

An unexpected and unwelcome consequence resulted from the findings and my relationship with the study sample. Although it is well known that interviewers find interviews stressful, the effects of the in-depth interview on the interviewer are largely ignored. Brannen (1988) believes that interviewers are often left to cope with the emotional after-effects of the interview as best they can, and suggests that lone interviewers are perhaps more vulnerable in this respect, because they are usually unable to seek support from others in the same predicament (Bar-On, 1996). Before commencing my research, my main PhD supervisor had suggested that I seek clinical supervision to help me cope with parents' emotional responses to the diagnosis but, because I had experienced parental distress in my clinical practice, I believed this was unnecessary. Contrary to my expectations, I found some of the interviews with parents upsetting, particularly when interviewing soon after diagnosis, and I re-visited the parents' distress during transcription of the audiotapes and during the final writing up phase of the research. For practical reasons and to ensure respondent confidentiality, I was unable to discuss my feelings with colleagues. This culminated in an intense feeling of sadness, which may have been partly due to the intense, isolating and stressful nature of writing up a doctoral study, but could also be attributed to the relationship I had developed with parents through my joint clinical and research roles. I would advise any researchers investigating emotive topics, particularly with participants with whom they had developed a clinical relationship, to obtain clinical supervision in addition to academic supervision.

Publication

The thesis was completed and successfully examined in 2000, after which I began to prepare papers for publication. At one stage in this process, a prestigious medical journal declined publication on the grounds that researching one's own clients was unethical, and one referee even went so far as to question the competence of my supervisors for allowing me to pursue 'flawed research'. A robust correspondence ensued, in which it was once again made clear that the study was not an evaluation, emphasizing the nature of qualitative enquiry and the attention that had been given to the trustworthiness of the findings. Although still declining to publish, the editor issued an unreserved apology for the allegation that had been made. After a further rejection from a different journal, the main paper describing my findings was accepted by a quality peer reviewed medical journal (Lowes *et al.*, 2004) and the findings have been generally well received by medical and nursing colleagues.

Case study 2: Researching one's own nursing students – Keith

This case study describes work in which I was both the research producer and the tutor for the group of students who participated in the study. Students are rarely identified as a vulnerable group in nursing research texts (Clark and McCann, 2005), but involvement in research as subjects can have significant outcomes for them and they are clearly in a position where their relationship with the researcher/educator is potentially one of unequal power. Hence the principles of respect and autonomy are of equal importance for students as they are for patients/clients.

Accessing the students' work for the purposes of research is an indirect way of studying them and raises issues about the power differential between researcher and researched. I will show how we strove to take this into consideration throughout the various stages in the project, in which my involvement as researcher was varied in terms of my own role *vis-à-vis* the students. To begin with I was a tutor and part of a team engaged in solving a particular educational problem, investigating students both directly and indirectly. Then I became a doctoral student as well as tutor, using my interactions with students in the course of my PhD investigation and, in collaboration with colleagues, conducting an experimental evaluation of a prototype educational system. As it became apparent that the work originating in my PhD had the potential for considerable expansion, the nature of the relationship changed yet again, but that is outside the scope of this present case study.

The emergent problem

In 1992 I was working with a biosciences team in a university-based school of nursing, teaching the application of health sciences and pharmacological principles to professional nursing practice. This included a module on medication dosage calculations. Routine assessments showed that significant numbers of students made dosage calculation errors, and continued to do so after completing the module. This problem was first described over 65 years ago (Faddis, 1939), and is still of concern today (Dean et al., 1995; Ridge et al., 1995; Lesar et al., 1997; Olsen et al., 1997; Taxis and Barber, 2003). Our bioscience team came to realize that we did not understand the origins of the problem and needed to initiate a programme of research to identify and describe the factors associated with students' difficulties. This would, of necessity, require us to work with clinical colleagues, pharmacy advisors and, most importantly, our own nursing students. We were concerned to accord respect to our students and to work with, rather than on them. This concern influenced the methodological choices that were made at all stages in the work.

Initial stages: researching students indirectly

The first phase was exploratory work, involving our students indirectly. The initial research group consisted of members of the biosciences team, who undertook a retrospective review of the errors recorded in the students' assessments from the medication dosage calculation module. This revealed three types: errors in performing arithmetic operations (e.g. converting fractions to decimal equivalents), computational errors (mistakes in long division, subtraction, etc.) and conceptual errors, i.e. failure to grasp the conceptual basis of the problem (Weeks, 2001). Many people in the population experience numeracy difficulties resulting in errors of the first two types and in this respect our students were no different from the UK population as a whole (Department of Education and Employment, 1999) and in nursing (Hutton, 1998; Weeks, 2001; Sabin, 2001). So we were not too surprised to find errors of the first two types, but we were perplexed by the prevalence of conceptual errors and the vague notions that many students had regarding the dosage problems they were attempting to solve. Although, at first sight, it might seem unproblematic for tutors to review a set of student assessments, in practice this gave us some concerns. That is, a fundamental tenet for educators practising within health care education programmes is that we have a professional and legal obligation to respond to assessment results that are related to the safety of the public.

Using our own students directly as informants

Once we had located the types of problem and the prevalence of conceptual errors we needed to gain further understanding of them from the students themselves. Engaging with our own students was essential, as it was necessary to undertake a detailed longitudinal study of their problems, a process that could not have been facilitated by studying students extrinsic to the organization. A series of individual interviews and focus group discussions with our students followed, where their opinions of problems with the learning process in our School were discussed with a core group of bioscience lecturers experienced within this domain of education and clinical practice. The data collected during these exchanges challenged our fundamental beliefs regarding theories of adult learning and the appropriateness of employing our traditional methods of education with novice learners. In summary, nursing students who had been taught medication dosage calculation skills through the methods we were using, stated that the process was: useful only for sitting written assessments, not relevant to the 'real world' of nursing, just numbers for numbers' sake, and used words such as 'prescribed' and 'dispensed dose' which held no real meaning. It was not useful as a preparation for undertaking dosage calculations in clinical practice as it failed to sensitize the students to the dosage problems seen there (Weeks, 2001). We recognized that, for the students to express such frank, challenging and illuminating views required a shift in the traditional teacher-dominated process, to a more flexible and constructivist centred relationship. To facilitate this it was necessary to promote active rather than passive student participation in the process, with an emphasis being placed on mutual respect and trust. Ultimately this could only be achieved over time and necessitated working directly with our students.

'Accidental' learning from my own students

The interviews revealed a great deal about the students' opinions of our teaching methods. However, for some time the actual nature of the problems being experienced by students eluded conceptualization. Students had frequently made comments like 'I can't see what you mean', which we had assumed to be a colloquialism, implying a lack of understanding. A defining event for me occurred during a chance meeting with a group of our students who had all been referred on the written assessment for this module. The meeting turned into an informal tutorial. The following is an extract from field notes taken at the time:

> I was working through word problems and the formula and equation used for calculating injection dosages.
>
> Keith: In this question we have: prescribed dose aminophilline 200 milligrams and dispensed dose 250 milligrams contained in a 10 millilitre ampoule ... how much aminophilline do we give? OK now what's the formula used to solve this problem?
>
> Becky, one of the students, told me that the word problems confused her, and that she 'couldn't get her head around things like prescribed dose', and 'what does 250 milligrams in 10 millilitres mean ... which bit goes where in the formula ... I just don't see what those words mean'. The other three students were nodding in agreement. Reflecting on a series of verbal evaluations of the dosage calculation lesson we had undertaken previously with students, I recalled that a common feature of many students' previous comments was:

'I can't *see* what he was saying ...'

'I just don't *see* what she was getting at' or

'No I still don't *see* it ...'

The repeated use of words associated with vision triggered the idea that this is what the students actually wished to convey. It was a question of actually visualizing the elements of the problem in concrete terms. The possibility that students might need to physically see or mentally visualize an object or artifact was to become pivotal to the future conceptualization of the problem. It led to the realization that the use of word problems, formulae and equations which were divorced from the real world inhibited the students' understanding of the dosage problems encountered in professional nursing practice (Weeks, 2001; Weeks et al., 2001). This was a totally unexpected serendipitous insight, and one example of the several instances which we experienced whilst working informally with students. Serendipity in research is defined as the emergence and recognition of contingencies not previously fully comprehended (Fine and Deegan, 1996). Thus involvement with our students gave access to territory which could not have been explored through any other means and our long involvement with them provided the prepared minds able to discern the patterns which led to our understanding of the nature of the problem. Ultimately this conceptualization framed all the work which followed, and subsequently underpinned a major action research project centred on the design, development and evaluation of a computer-based Authentic World® Medication Dosage Calculation program, part of which formed the basis for my doctoral thesis.

Involving students directly in action research and experimental evaluation

The first step was the design and evaluation of a prototype learning program. By this time I had registered the study for my PhD, which added a layer of complexity to my relationship with the students who were to be involved in this phase of the work. My doctoral studies had to be undertaken on a part-time basis since, like many lecturers in nursing, I had no access to external funding, although I received some support from my employing organization. In this phase of the work the research team consisted of me, a fellow lecturer and a principal pharmacist. Our nursing students took part in the design of the program by consistently evaluating the emerging construction of a program that was specifically designed to address the problems identified and operationalized during our previous collaborative work. This collaboration provided critical feedback during the iterative process undertaken during the program's development. Production of the prototype (Weeks, 2001) was followed by its evaluation. For this a cross-over experimental approach was selected in order to determine the relationship between exposure to the prototype program and the prevalence of errors.

Nursing research has been much criticized for the production of vague and inconclusive results. Watson (2003) considers that scientific methods are the only credible way forward for nursing research. The ideal design for attributing an outcome to an intervention, as demanded by this case, is the classic or true experiment originating in the natural sciences. Educational research, which has been located on the boundary between the natural and human sciences, has a history of failure in the application of the experimental paradigm to educational problems, largely due to the difficulty of controlling the conditions of experiments outside strict laboratory conditions and the variability and autonomy of the research subjects (teachers and learners). Despite the criticisms that have been levelled at experimental research in nursing, we were convinced that an experimental approach could be used to produce meaningful data on the effectiveness of the prototype, whilst at the same time respecting the rights of the subjects as persons and student nurses and taking account of our relationship with them as their tutors.

It was necessary to design the evaluation so that we could be clear about the relationship between interventions and outcome (internal validity) and generalizability of the findings (external validity). These conditions become even more important, as in our case when the researcher has close contact with the research subjects and interest in the research field. External validity is particularly contentious under these circumstances. Subsequently we drew on the seminal work of Campbell and Stanley (1963) to guide the design. As illustrated in Figure 10.1 we employed a cross-over or repeat measure experimental design. This is an especially powerful method of ensuring equivalence between the groups being compared, i.e. of controlling all extraneous subject characteristics, as each subject effectively acts as his/her own control.

Using the population of pre-registration diploma students following the Foundation Programme, we randomly selected a 40 per cent sample ($n = 44$) and randomly assigned 22 students to each of the two experimental groups. A full explanation of the rationale and scope of the research programme was provided and written informed consent gained from each participant. We had suspected that given the vast literature on mathaphobia or maths avoidance that a potentially large proportion of the available population of students ($N = 110$) would decline to take part in the study. However, to our surprise the entire cohort of students volunteered for inclusion, and although anecdotal it emerged from a general discussion with the group that dosage calculations represented a major fear for a very large percentage of these students, which prompted them to take all opportunities to develop this skill.

Table 10.1 Features of the cross-over experimental design

Phase and week	Group and treatment	Group and treatment
Phase 1 Week 1	*Computer laboratory* Group X (22 subjects) Authentic World learning environment (90-minute exposure)	*Classroom* Group Y (22 subjects) Didactic transmission method (90-minute exposure)
Phase 1 Week 3	Group X (22 subjects) Authentic World learning environment (90-minute exposure)	Group Y (22 subjects) Teacher led tutorial (90-minute exposure)
Phase 1 Week 4	30-point written medication dosage calculation assessment	
Phase 2 Week 5	*Classroom* Group X (22 subjects) Didactic transmission method (90-minute exposure)	*Computer laboratory* Group Y (22 subjects) Authentic World learning environment (90-minute exposure)
Phase 2 Week 7	Group X (22 subjects) Teacher led tutorial (90-minute exposure)	Group Y (22 subjects) Authentic World learning environment (90-minute exposure)
Phase 2 Week 8	30-point written medication dosage calculation assessment	

Methodological issues

Campbell and Stanley (1963) and Cook and Campbell (1979) identified 12 conditions that must be satisfied before internal validity can be assumed, and four threats to external validity. A full analysis of how the identified threats to internal and external validity were acknowledged and, where possible, controlled is provided elsewhere (Weeks, 2001). Here we will focus on those features salient to engaging one's own students in the research process. The most important of these is the question of potential bias caused by the relationship between the investigator and the participants. In this case, I was the originator of the Authentic World program, which was being evaluated, as well as being a PhD student with an interest in producing a successful thesis and the tutor for these students. I acknowledged the possibility for bias in terms of the allocation of participants to groups, the administration of the interventions and the assessment of the outcome. To address this, administration of both the Authentic World program and the traditional didactic lesson were undertaken by lecturers with appropriate experience but who were independent of the design and development team. Subsequent assessment and analysis of student performance was based on rigorous application of fully operationalized definitions of the three error types previously described, by independent lecturers and practitioners, and cross-referenced by myself for accuracy.

In terms of research design it was tempting to select the classical experimental design, with one experimental group (sole exposure to the Authentic World environment) and one control group (sole exposure to the didactic transmission lesson). This design would have eliminated the potential for multiple-treatment interference, a threat to external validity which is present when the same participants are used repeatedly for two or more treatments and the effects of the previous treatments are not erasable. However, our plan was to follow a sub-sample of participants into clinical practice to discover if the level of performance achieved during the experiment transferred into the clinical setting. We were sufficiently convinced, by our exploratory work, of the benefits of using the prototype to predict that those who had been exposed to it would do much better in their subsequent practice and those who had not been exposed would continue to have their original difficulties. We were not prepared to prejudice students' development by undertaking a clinical assessment which could be a very negative experience for the student, and which could impact on their future progress in this key skill. For this reason, whilst acknowledging the limitations described by Fleiss (1986) we selected the cross-over design in which all students would be exposed to both traditional teaching and the new learning programme.

On completion of the experiment we found that the Authentic World learning environment eliminated all conceptual errors; there was a highly significant reduction in other error types and student performance transferred to practice settings. The results of the work have been widely disseminated at national and international conferences and have been reported elsewhere (Weeks, 2001). Ultimately the study has formed the basis for increasingly widespread change in educational practice and an ongoing programme of international post-doctoral research. Since completion of the original research an advanced version of the prototype Authentic World® medication dosage calculation learning environment has been developed (see www.authenticworld.com for an animated illustration). This account of its early development has, we hope, demonstrated how firm foundations can be created through close involvement of students from the outset and also illuminated some of the particular issues which need to be addressed.

Discussion

Together, these two case studies bring to light several of the interactions described in Part I of this book, which shape nursing research involving those with whom the researchers have a caring or educational relationship. They also demonstrate the strengths and challenges of working in this way, which have to be carefully balanced by those who propose to adopt this strategy.

Intersection of professional and research ethics

Both the studies were strongly influenced by the nursing professional discourse, which embodies ethical standards to be observed with all research subjects. This created the framework for their work involving clients both directly and indirectly. In addition to this, the researchers' involvement with the subjects in a professional capacity created a personal agenda based on their intimate knowledge of the subjects' worlds and the likely consequences for them of participation in the planned research. This influenced the design of the study in both cases.

Steering a course through diverse disciplinary paradigms

The views of influential stakeholders about the scientific desirability of working with one's own clients entered many discussions. So the form and progress of both projects were shaped by these intersecting factors and the varied views within competing discourses of the advisability of research with previously known subjects. The biomedical research paradigm was strongly present in the context of Lesley's study, where she was obliged to counter any propensity for bias by including the nearest thing she could find to a control group (i.e. patients whose main carer was not Lesley but a colleague) and the mistaken but frequently held assumption that she was evaluating her practice and thus required such a control group for that purpose. During her attempts to publish the result, this assumption resurfaced and led to an almost libellous attack on the quality of the work. Happily, this view was confined to a single editorial board which retracted its statement. Whether this resulted from conviction that a mistake had been made or fear of litigation can never be known. In Keith's study the same scientific basis for experimental design was filtered through the educational research tradition, in which the realities of experimentation using autonomous subjects are better appreciated. He and his colleagues saw this as a highly desirable means of producing meaningful evaluation data to enable them to progress their prototype learning environment and went against the grain of much nursing research which decries the use of experimentation. Their preferred design was modified as a result of their appreciation of the impact it might have on the progress of the students who participated.

Conclusions

Although research involving one's own clients or students brings a number of dilemmas, both case studies include strategies for resolving them and reveal benefits resulting from intimate knowledge of the study phenomena. We concur with Whyte (1992), believing that the advantages of the dual role far outweigh the disadvantages. In the first place, clients or students can be in the best possible position to influence certain kinds of research. They may be the only source from which the required data can be generated, or the only people who can identify the true nature of the problem. As in Keith's study, the researcher's association with them has the potential to create the prepared mind, capable of making sense of apparently unconnected nuances within the research environment and leading to the unexpected (or serendipitous) insights that commonly run counter to previous expectations. Ultimately all researchers who engage their clients and students in the research process must strike a balance between capitalizing on the advantages and dealing with the threats of working in this way.

Acknowledgements

Lesley Lowes's doctoral study was supported by a personal bursary from the Wales Office of Research and Development for Health and Social Care (WORD).

References

Ashworth, P. (1987) *Adequacy of Description: The Validity of Qualitative Findings in Education Management*, Sheffield: Sheffield City Polytechnic, Department of Education Management.

Bar-On, D. (1996) 'Ethical issues in biographical interviews and analysis', in R. Josselson (ed.) *Ethics and Process in the Narrative Study of Lives*, Thousand Oaks, CA: Sage Publications.

Bowler, I. (1997) 'Problems with interviewing: experiences with service providers and clients', in G. Miller and R. Dingwall (eds) *Context and Method in Qualitative Research*, London: Sage Publications.

Brannen, J. (1988) 'The study of sensitive subjects', *Sociological Review*, 36, 552–63.

Campbell, D. and Stanley, J. (1963) 'Experimental and quasi-experimental designs for research and teaching', in N. Gage (ed.) *Handbook on Teaching*, Chicago, IL: Rand McNally.

Campbell, T. (1999) 'Feelings of oncology patients about being nursed in protective isolation as a consequence of cancer chemotherapy treatment', *Journal of Advanced Nursing*, 30, 439–47.

Clark, E. and McCann, T.V. (2005) 'Researching students: An ethical dilemma', *Nurse Researcher*, 12, 42–50.

Cook, T. and Campbell, D. (1979) *Quasi-Experimentation: Design and Analysis Issues for Field Settings*, Boston, MA: Houghton Mifflin.

Dean, B., Allan, E., Barber, N. and Barker, K. (1995) 'Comparison of medication errors in an American and a British hospital', *American Journal of Health-System Pharmacy*, 52, 2543–9.

Department of Education and Employment (1999) *The Moser Report: A Fresh Start: Improving Literacy and Numeracy*, London: DofEE.

Faddis, M. (1939) 'Eliminating errors in medication', *American Journal of Nursing*, 39, 1217.

Fine, G.A. and Deegan, J.G. (1996) 'Three principles of serendipity: insight, chance and discovery in qualitative research', *International Journal of Qualitative Studies in Education*, 9, 434–47.

Fleiss, J.L. (1986) *The Design and Analysis of Clinical Experiments*, New York: John Wiley and Sons.

Guba, E.G. (1981) 'Criteria for assessing the trustworthiness of naturalistic inquiries', *Education Communication Technology Journal*, 29, 75–91.

Hutton, B.M. (1998) 'Nursing mathematics: the importance of application', *Nursing Standard* 13, 35–8.

Koch, T. (1996) 'Implementation of a hermeneutic inquiry in nursing: philosophy, rigour and representation', *Journal of Advanced Nursing*, 24, 174–84.

Lesar, T., Briceland, L. and Stein, D. (1997) 'Factors related to errors in medication prescribing', *Journal of American Medical Association*, 277, 312–17.

Long, S. (1997) 'Being together as a family', *Paediatric Nursing*, 9, 25–8.

Lowes, L. (2000) 'Newly diagnosed childhood diabetes: parents' experience of home management and coping over the first year', Unpublished PhD Thesis, Nursing, Health and Social Care Research Centre, School of Nursing and Midwifery Studies. Cardiff: University of Wales College of Medicine.

Lowes, L., Gregory, J.W. and Lyne, P. (2005) 'Newly diagnosed childhood diabetes: a psychosocial transition for parents?', *Journal of Advanced Nursing*, 50, 253–61.

Lowes, L., Lyne, P. and Gregory, J.W. (2004) 'Childhood diabetes: parents' experience of home management and the first year following diagnosis', *Diabetic Medicine*, 21, 531–8.

Lyon, J. and Walker, C. (eds) (1997) *Ethical Issues*, Edinburgh: Churchill Livingstone.

May, K.M. (1991) 'Interview techniques in qualitative research: Concerns and challenges', in J.M. Morse (ed.) *Qualitative Nursing Research: A Contemporary Dialogue*, Newbury Park, CA: Sage Publications.

Olsen, P., Lorentzen, H., Thomsen, K. and Fogtmann, A. (1997) 'Fejlmedicinering pa en borneafdeling' [Medication errors in a pediatric department]. [in Danish]. *Ugeskrift for Laeger*, 159, 2392–5.

Ridge, K.W., Jenkins, D.B., Noyce, P. and Barber, N.D. (1995) 'Medication errors during hospital drug rounds', *Quality in Health Care*, 4, 240–3.

Rodgers, B.L. and Cowles, K.C. (1993) 'The qualitative research audit trail: a complex collection of documentation', *Research in Nursing and Health*, 16, 219–26.

Sabin, M. (2001) *Competence in Practice Based Calculation: Issues for Nursing Education: A Critical Review of the Literature*, London, LTSN.

Streubert, H.J. (1995) 'Philosophical dimensions of qualitative research', in H.J. Streubert and D.R. Carpenter (eds) *Qualitative Research in Nursing: Advancing the Humanistic Imperative*, Philadelphia, PA: J.B. Lippincott.

Taxis, K. and Barber, N. (2003) 'Ethnographic study of incidence and severity of intravenous drug errors', *British Medical Journal* 326, 684.

Van Stuijvenberg, M., Suur, M.H., De Vos, S., Tjiang, G.C.H., Steyerberg, E.W., Derksen-Lubsen, G. and Moll, H.A. (1998) 'Informed consent, parental awareness and reasons for participating in a randomised controlled trial', *Archives of Disease in Childhood*, 79, 120–5.

Watson, R. (2003) Editorial, *Journal of Advanced Nursing*, 43, 219–20.

Weeks, K.W. (2001) 'Setting a foundation for the development of medication dosage calculation problem solving skills among novice nursing students. The role of constructivist learning approaches and a computer based "Authentic World" learning environment', Unpublished PhD Thesis, University of Glamorgan.

Weeks, K.W., Lyne, P., Mosely, L. and Torrance, C. (2001) 'The strive for clinical effectiveness in medication dosage calculation problem solving skills: the role of constructivist theory in the design of a computer-based "authentic world" learning environment', *Clinical Effectiveness in Nursing*, 5, 18–25.

Whyte, D.A. (1992) 'A family nursing approach to the care of a child with a chronic illness', *Journal of Advanced Nursing*, 17, 317–27.

Relationship with the data (analysis)

Davina Allen and Patricia Lyne

Introduction

In Part I we described how several discourses interact to shape the research undertaken by nurses and midwives. These are of a relatively high order, being common to whole professional and social groups. However, there are further layers of complexity to be explored. Within and running across these major groupings are other sets of ideas and ways of thinking that distinguish smaller groupings which share social and educational influences. In this chapter we will consider how such influences affect the way that nurse researchers engage in the processes of converting raw data, from whatever source, into answers to their research questions, i.e. the analysis and subsequent interpretation of the data.

One reason for attempting this is to challenge the view that there is a single unified body of work that can lay legitimate claim to the title 'nursing research'. Another is to help increase mutual respect and understanding between the many different research groups making up this broad field. The third, and perhaps the most practically important one, is to demonstrate the value of reflection on our journeys into research careers. We believe that it is important to be aware, at any stage, of the factors that have shaped our present situation and to place them in a wider context. This is of particular importance in terms of the way we view the relationship between the data generated by our studies and the meaning derived from our interpretation of those data.

We do not intend to replay any of the existing debates about quantitative and qualitative methods. At an early stage in the research career any nurse will be aware that these have been presented extensively, some might say *ad nauseam* (Blaxter *et al.*, 2001) and, in some cases, the impression is of two opposing camps of researchers, with very little appreciation of the skills or values of the other. There is also a tendency for debates about this paradigm conflict to become inextricably linked with clashes over professional power and gender issues, some of which are illustrated in other case studies in this book. Rather, through an exploration of two contrasting research trajectories, we will try to illustrate what produces an individual's orientation to data handling. We will argue that insight into the range and variety of individual approaches promotes creativity in research and is helpful in dealing with many of the issues which are raised in Part II of this book.

Case study 1: Patricia

My route into nursing research has been, to say the least, unconventional. In treating this trajectory as a case study I will focus on those elements which have influenced my present appreciation of ways of describing the world, i.e. our observations and how we analyse and interpret them.

The obvious starting point for me is a vivid memory of being 'switched on' to science at the age of 15. This is a very long time ago now and my memories of school are few and far between, but this one stands out with remarkable clarity. If I enjoyed any subject it was maths, for which I had some facility, and physics was my second preference. I was ordinarily somewhat dismissive of biology, but on this particular day I can remember the exact classroom in which a biology lesson took place, the fine, sunny day, a picture (cypresses by Van Gogh) on the wall beside the blackboard and the name of the teacher. She was not a particularly good teacher and we did not usually pay much attention, but in this lesson she was trying to explain to us something called the Krebs cycle, which seemed incredibly boring until she said 'and the same system powers all kinds of plants and animals'. This really hit me between the eyes. To think that it was possible to understand some (invisible) engine which was the source of all living activity seemed to me to be a truly wonderful thing and something that I wanted to know more about.

However, with no tradition of university education in the family and the need to earn a living I left school the following year. The germ of scientific interest made me resist working in the mill, the most usual employment in our town, and seek out the nearest thing to science. This was a local pharmaceutical firm, where I became a lab assistant, not learning much actual science but getting a good grounding in laboratory practice. My job included quality control on batches of drugs and I became very aware that accuracy and precision in measurement could reveal things of importance in the real world.

I had the great good fortune to be encouraged by the senior pharmacist who made it possible for me to do A levels by day release and eventually get into university to study Biochemistry, first as an undergraduate and then, rather to my surprise, as a doctoral student. I find it interesting to reflect that there was no component of our undergraduate course with the label 'methodology' or 'research'. We absorbed the philosophy of science, experimental design, laboratory techniques and data analysis through practical experience.

A major tenet of laboratory experimentation is that of control. At the simplest, two systems are set up in which all conditions are identical. Then something is done or added to one system but not the other and the results are compared. Any resultant differences between the control and the experimental systems are attributed to the way the experimental system has been treated. This is, in effect, a procedure for eliminating all other possible explanations for whatever may be observed. I spent a lot of time working with a particular purified enzyme to investigate its mode of action and the conditions necessary for this action. This involved setting up elaborate controlled experiments with perhaps ten or 12 reaction vessels that were all identical before receiving varied experimental treatments. This enabled us to determine what the enzyme did to its substrate, what intermediates were formed and what other factors were involved. The numerical data produced showed, for example, how fast the enzyme worked when exposed to different environmental conditions, such as the pH (degree of acidity). The interpretation was that, under the conditions of the experiment, the enzyme converted its substrate to the product that was being measured most rapidly at pH 7.2, assuming that there were no systematic differences between the control and experimental systems. This may not sound a very exciting piece of information, but in the overall scheme of things, our understanding of the way that living cells operate is built up of small pieces of knowledge such as this. The careful interpretation is important, because it expresses exactly what can be deduced from the available data.

Throughout this period I was gradually becoming a part of a scientific community whose members shared a common approach to investigation which was based on the development of sophisticated instrumentation and its use in elegant experimental studies. This was the era when the mechanisms of DNA replication and transcription were being elucidated. Better techniques for isolating, purifying and studying enzymes were being developed. It is difficult to convey the sense of excitement in that community at that time. There was a sense that the unknown was becoming knowable. As a (junior) insider in this community I shared this excitement and also observed the arguments about what the emergent data revealed.

During my undergraduate studies I gradually learnt more about the topic that had originally inspired me, the Krebs cycle. Although we did not formally study 'research' we were instructed in the history of how our current knowledge had been developed. We were shown how, over a period of some five years, H.A. Krebs had brought together many pieces of a jigsaw of knowledge concerning the cellular events leading to the liberation of useful energy from foodstuffs (i.e. cellular respiration). Finally he himself discovered a reaction which made sense of all the others and allowed him to propose the cyclic nature of the respiratory process (Krebs et al., 1938).

My good luck continued when, after completing my PhD, I was able to spend three years in Oxford working in Krebs' laboratory. The first research presentation I ever gave was shortly after arriving there, with Krebs himself in the middle of the front row. The combination of a pronounced Yorkshire accent and sheer terror made me totally incomprehensible to most of the audience. However, HAK turned out to be very approachable, always ready to support young researchers and to imbue his sense of the importance of accurate observation. This was where I learnt most about experimental design, good technique and, above all, the sense that numbers could really tell you something if you treated them properly.

The attitude of scientists to qualitative observations at that time was that they were important and a necessary precursor to quantification. For example, Krebs describes how he discovered that, in living muscle tissue, two key metabolites combine to produce citric acid, which provided a possible mechanism for the operation of the respiratory cycle. At this stage, however, he notes that the information was 'only qualitative' (Krebs, 1981) and it was necessary to find out if the rates at which these reactions occurred were sufficient to support the cyclic hypothesis (i.e. to quantify the phenomenon). In other words, there were no numerical data to describe how these metabolites interact. This conceptualization of qualitative information pervaded and still pervades the scientific community and, by extension, is influential in the education of medical students. It refers to observations that cannot be defined in numerical terms. It is a very different concept from that of qualitative social science and nursing, which perhaps goes some way to explaining the sterility of the paradigm debates. Maybe it is important that we have a better understanding of these differences so that discussion of the relative contributions of numerical and non-numerical data can be more fruitful.

After several happy and productive years in academic biochemistry circumstances made it necessary for me to suspend my career for over ten years, during which I worked as a volunteer in a hospice. When the time came to resume full-time work, my life experiences had inclined me towards a different career and instead of returning to university as a lecturer I embarked upon nurse training, subsequently working in accident and emergency and terminal care.

As a nurse I found myself exposed to a range of new and very different research problems. At first I thought that application of the familiar scientific methods would solve them. These depend on the existence of accurate measurement methods which allow the degree of error to be known, their use with homogeneous populations and the employment of probabilistic techniques to produce statistics which are then capable of interpretation. Fundamental to this approach is that numerical measurements are treated according to the principles of mathematics, and that the resultant interpretation, through which their meaning is derived, rests firmly or solely on the correct manipulation of the numerical data.

I soon found that there were many problems that could not be addressed in this way. When starting to explore the research base of nursing, the first group that I encountered were nurses with backgrounds in psychology. I found their approach to measurement quite surprising. They appeared to me to be trying to measure things that you could not pin down or put through a machine, and I was even more surprised to find that they used numbers that, in my opinion, were not real in that they did not possess the properties of numbers which are necessary for the performance of arithmetic operations (Lyne, 1994). After a time, however, I understood that this compromise might be necessary, because so many of the phenomena of interest to nursing were not amenable to measurement in the way that was familiar to me. I was reminded that different professions regard numbers in different ways. There is an old joke, of which I have been unable to discover the origin, although it is generally told by scientists and engineers. When asked 'what is two plus two?', an accountant will say that this makes exactly four, a scientist will say that after careful investigation there is evidence that the answer lies somewhere between three and five, but a psychologist will ask you why you need to know the answer to that question.

Soon I came across nurse researchers grounded in other social science disciplines who, to my horror, were not attempting to measure anything at all and I had to revise my ideas even further. So began a lifelong interest in methods, attempting to discover the best and most rigorous ways to answer the difficult questions posed in nursing research. Along the way I have investigated a range of approaches to data generation and the subsequent handling and analysis of the data. At first I was extremely sceptical about non-numerical data. But as I began to read and take instruction around what I learnt to call qualitative inquiry I appreciated the contextualized nature of this enterprise and the nature of data analysis and interpretation. I could appreciate that the elements of the whole process are interactive in a way that differs markedly from the scientific enterprise, where analysis of the data follows the tenets of mathematical theory and the research is designed to eliminate any influence from the researcher, who remains detached from the process. The meaning of the end product is that the data have been processed through this system and produced a certain answer, which is interpreted in that light. I learnt that in qualitative research the analysis is an entirely different process, in which the researcher is intimately involved, but, in the same way, the meaning of the end product is that the data have been subjected to clearly described processes, producing findings to be interpreted in that light. I also came to realize that, to be done to the highest standard, this is a very challenging enterprise, requiring minute attention to detail and considerable intellectual rigour.

In clinical practice I came to realize that there was very little evidence on which to base our nursing decisions. This was brought into sharp focus for me when caring for people who had difficult wounds as a result of advanced cancer, particularly fungating and ulcerating malignant lesions (Ivetic and Lyne, 1990). I tried very hard to buy out some time to carry out research in this area, but with no avail. The time was not right, but I am glad to know that nurse researchers have now been able to carry out funded work in this area and apply a new way of thinking to the study of the effectiveness of dressings for this distressing condition (Browne et al., 2003). My continuing interest in research led me to take up a part-time research and clinical post and then to return to education. This coincided with the emergence of the evidence-based health care movement and led me down the path of becoming a methodologist.

I have developed a particular interest in the nature of evidence and how it is appraised and used in practice. During the earlier stages of this career I constantly found myself frustrated by the overpowering influence of professional agenda on the freedom of aspirant researchers. I had always seen research problems in isolation from any political context (except, of course, where there were funding questions). By and large, what was of importance was the significance and interest of the research topic and the potential findings. But as I increasingly worked with people who were just beginning their research careers I observed that they were constantly encountering closed doors, or rather, no go areas which were barred for a number of reasons: resources; the need to produce a 'useful' result; the potential implications of the findings for others and the relationship of the research to the professional and educational climate of the day. On the other hand, I often found that the impetus for the research was not detached interest, but sprang from a desire to 'prove' that a service was doing a good job, or even to justify the need for a particular nursing role. I had to ask questions such as: 'What if the study shows that this service is doing no good at all?' to an amazed student who had never entertained this possibility. The view that I have developed around data analysis stems from this belief, that as researchers we have a duty to put before the users of research results whose meaning is entirely clear whatever their degree of uncertainty.

Case study 2: Davina

My first exposure to research and research methods was as an A level sociology student. Sociology is a multi-paradigmatic discipline; different theories exist to explain social phenomena and these in turn point to different methods of data collection. One of the most compelling illustrations of this overall point is in the case of the sociological study of suicide where competing definitions of the nature of the problem lead to quite different conclusions as to the appropriate approach to its study.

Durkheim's study of suicide is a sociological classic (Durkheim, 1952). First published in 1897, it is seen by many as a model of social research (Selvin, 1965). Durkheim believed that if sociology was to be given the same intellectual status as a discipline as the natural sciences, then, like them, it ought to be capable of formulating universal laws which explain its operation and effects. For Durkheim, society was more than the sum of its parts; it exercised power and influence over individual action and behaviour. What better way to prove this point than to demonstrate that suicide, the most individual of all acts, is socially determined? In order to prove his hypothesis Durkheim collated suicide statistics from different societies and different social groups and was able to demonstrate that within single societies the rate of suicide remains remarkably consistent over time and that different societies and different groups within the same society have different suicide rates. Durkheim endeavoured to explain his findings in terms of a theory of social integration. He argued that suicide rates are highest in those social groups where integration is very low or very high. In the former there are few social ties and suicide arises because of excessive individualism; in the latter the individual is so totally immersed in the life of a group that as an individual they have no value. 'Anomic suicide' occurs at times when there is a break down in the normal social order through which individual behaviours are regulated.

The classic alterative to this perspective is presented by Douglas (Douglas, 1967) who criticizes Durkheim for assuming that society influences suicide in a uni-directional fashion, leaving no scope for consideration of how social reality is actively created by social actors in circumstances which have meaning for them. Douglas directs attention to the social construction of the suicide statistics on which Durkheim's analysis depends and asks how it is that certain acts come to be interpreted as suicide and not others? He points to wide variation in the practices of coroners in Western society in certifying a death as a suicide and also points to the actions of individuals in arranging and framing the circumstances of their death so that it is interpreted in one way rather than another. Douglas does not deny that suicide is socially patterned, but points to the interpretative practices through which acts come to be defined as such, rather than assuming they can be explained solely as the result of social forces.

Exposure to this case study had a profound effect in highlighting the complexity of studying social life and in particular the value of synthesizing different approaches. Giddens (1977) suggests how this might be achieved in the study of suicide, but the general observation holds true for any substantive area of concern. The case also revealed to me in powerful ways the social processes through which statistics are constructed and the need for methodological transparency in the representation of social 'reality'.

Whilst the contested nature of knowledge is inherent to the discipline of sociology, it was only in the latter part of the course that this was explicitly linked to the research endeavour. The production of sociological knowledge was to constitute a compulsory question in our final examination and was given a particular emphasis over and above the substantive topics studied in the rest of the syllabus. We considered in some detail the relationship between ontology (different propositions about what is), epistemology (different techniques for establishing what can be accepted as real), methodology (the logic of inquiry) and methods (techniques for data collection). We learnt that no method was inherently superior but that having adopted a particular ontological and epistemological stand point one was more likely to be drawn to some methods rather than others. What was of utmost importance was the congruence between these different elements of a given study.

Following my A levels I commenced nurse training, where I found that the world view I had developed over the previous two years jarred with that which was required to get by as student nurse. The exploration of alternative explanations for clinical scenarios does little to endear colleagues to you in the real world of practice where one world view dominates all others and the emphasis is on action and getting through the work. Moreover, I have always had a preference for understanding through exploring how things actually happen rather than problem solving through the application of algorithms and formulae and at the time it was the latter that was the predominant educational ethos. Throughout my nursing career, I felt most comfortable in the mental health context, where competing explanations for mental ill health seemed to have created a greater preparedness to explore alternative approaches and a more critical approach to clinical work. Had I not made the decision to return to full-time education, I would almost certainly have followed this as a career path.

After five years in nursing, I was disenchanted with the work, finding the compromises required in the workplace difficult to reconcile with my own values. I returned to full-time education to study for a degree in sociology. Here my exposure to alternate approaches to the study of social life was further extended by the requirement to undertake courses in additional (subsidiary) subjects. In addition to sociology, I also studied social policy and psychology which offered new layers of understanding. These came together in my third year dissertation topic in which I studied nursing morale. Against a policy context of concern over recruitment and retention and partly driven by my own biography I undertook a questionnaire survey of nurses working in two different hospitals in order to examine sources of work satisfaction and dissatisfaction. The study was small scale and used very simple descriptive statistics. Nevertheless it revealed commonalities which pointed to dissatisfaction residing in features of the workplace rather than in the characteristics of nursing work. I used these findings as a starting point for developing a sociological critique of psychological models of occupational stress where the onus is on the individual to seek solutions to the problem rather than this being the responsibility of health service organizations.

Shortly after graduating I was employed as a research assistant working with Dr David Hughes on a 12 month policy-oriented study which entailed reviewing UK and North American ethnographic studies of health care work (Hughes and Allen, 1993b). The aim of the review was to examine research on workplace cultures and the division of labour to consider the lessons that could be learnt for issues of organizational governance. This project was highly influential in shaping my intellectual mindset and approach to data analysis. It exposed me to sociological studies of health care settings and ethnography for the first time. This enabled me to stand back from the world with which I was so familiar and see it with fresh eyes through an alternative interpretative lens. This had the effect of unsettling so much of what I had hitherto taken for granted and contributed to my understanding of some of the elements of health care work which I had found so difficult. Furthermore, because I was so familiar with the social worlds the sociologists sought to describe I felt well placed to critique the analyses offered. The summaries I made of the studies reviewed are littered with my own commentary on the text and revealed to me the value of insider knowledge in informing any analysis.

Reviewing a body of work in this way also highlighted the subtle differences in approaches to analysis and representation which are subsumed by the term 'ethnography'. The studies reviewed ranged from broadly focused descriptive monographs of health care settings where the emphasis was on evoking an overall picture of a work place culture (Fairhurst, 1971) to more detailed analyses of particular health care practices, such as managing medical mistakes (Bosk, 1979) or patterns of time in hospital life (Zerubavel, 1979). The studies also varied in their modes of representation. Some were predominantly narrative in style with field data and analysis seamlessly interwoven. In such cases the persuasiveness of the account was derived from the richness of the description and the extent to which the different elements of the story hung together in ways which rang true. In others, authors maintained a clear distinction between the data and the analysis (Dingwall, 1977) allowing the reader to judge the validity of the account according to the degree of fit between the two. Whilst the different approaches had their merits, my personal preference was for contextualized but focused studies in which the relationship between data and analysis was readily apparent.

The ethnographic review was followed by a pilot study, funded by South East Thames Regional Health Authority (SETRHA), which explored the opportunities for nursing role development as a result of the junior doctors' hours initiative (Hughes and Allen, 1993a). For this study we developed a survey instrument which produced quantitative and qualitative data. The quantitative materials were analyzed using SPSS and the qualitative materials were transcribed and categorized thematically. The two elements of the study were then considered together to build up an overview of health care providers' different attitudes to role change. The qualitative data provided important contextual information which shaped analysis of the quantitative materials; the latter had revealed interesting patterns and relationships but could tell us little about the underlying reasons for the responses given. Whilst the study achieved its aims as far as the Health Authority was concerned, the data were unable to generate the same depth of understanding which had characterized many of the ethnographic studies I had previously reviewed. Furthermore, funded as it was by the Health Authority, it was very much driven by a policy agenda about which I was not uncritical.

An opportunity to ameliorate this situation came in 1993 when I was fortunate enough to be awarded a UK Department of Health PhD studentship to undertake ethnographic research into the social processes through which nurses negotiated their work roles in daily practice. I was registered in a sociology department and supervised by a sociologist and a nurse. Like the SETRHA study I took the junior doctors' hours initiative and its implications for nursing roles as the policy context for the research, but my approach was very different. I was strongly influenced by the year spent reviewing the ethnographic literature where the Chicago School of Sociology – and Strauss et al.'s negotiated order perspective (Strauss et al., 1963) – had been particularly influential in shaping qualitative studies of healthcare contexts. As a result of my clinical experiences I was drawn to a perspective which acknowledged the situated character of nursing practice and the contextual factors which fashion its shape and form. Nevertheless, I had felt a degree of dissatisfaction with the lack of naturally occurring data that was made available to the reader in early negotiated order research, as compared to some of the ethnomethodologically oriented work to which I had been exposed (Dingwall, 1977). I was also keen to build into my approach an acknowledgement of the structures (particular gender) within which nurses worked. The negotiated order perspective, whilst acknowledging the constraints on social action, on the whole does not foreground this in the analysis. In the event my approach to my analysis was a synthesis of these different perspectives.

Whilst I recognized the value of my insider knowledge in undertaking a study of this kind, I was also concerned to retain a scholarly distance from a social world with which I was already familiar. I decided that one way in which I could achieve this goal would be by keeping the data and the analysis quite distinct. Accordingly, I adopted a behavioural approach to field notes in which I made literal descriptions of my observations, keeping this separate from my interpretations of their significance. Having a clear sense of the kind of analysis one wishes to pursue at an early stage in the research project is vital, as this critically influences the nature of the data generated. This is as true within a single method as it is where the choice may be between different methods.

The study combined observations with interviews and proved to be highly significant in shaping my orientation to the analysis of interview data. My findings revealed to me the discrepancy between what people say in interviews and what they do in practice and how the interview, as a locally situated social encounter in which 'identity work' is taking place, shapes the accounts that are produced. I was made aware of my own role as a data generator and the need to take this into account in my approach to the analysis (Allen, 2004).

Throughout the course of my PhD I reviewed a range of related literature and became very attracted to the methodological rigour and transparency which appeared to be offered by discourse and conversational analytic approaches. Indeed, I attended one supervision having just read Gilbert and Mulkay's (1984) wonderful study of scientific practice, and informed my supervisors that it was my intention to explore the literature on discourse and conversation analysis before I commenced writing up my thesis. Their response to this proposition was unequivocal: 'You have undertaken a classic ethnography of professional work and should just get on and write it up in those terms'. I was a bit taken aback by both the message and the brusqueness of its mode of delivery, but it was sound advice. Whilst the discourse and conversation analytic literature was a extension of the broadly ethnomethodological paradigm I had adopted, if that was the kind of analysis that I wished to undertake, then I should have generated data of a rather different kind. Maybe, also, my supervisors interpreted this as evidence of a reluctance to get on with the challenging job of data analysis. Having successful completed my PhD I have since had an opportunity to indulge my interests in this area. For this I re-transcribed and re-analysed data in order to explore the role of atrocity stories in the social construction of nurses' boundaries with medicine (Allen, 2001). Such work has an intrinsic appeal, as it is fine-grained, and rigorous. Nevertheless, its practical application is less immediate and given my ethnographic roots, I still feel the need for sufficient detail on the wider ethnographic context in studies of this kind. However, in analysing my interview data using a discourse analytic approach I was also made aware of the rhetorical resources and repertoires that are acquired as part of becoming a member of a particular social group which shape the way in which we narrate our experiences. This has strengthened my discomfiture about the capacity of interviews to provide unmediated access to psychological process or lived experiences. Whilst I think interviews are a useful tool in the researcher's toolkit, the data they generate and one's approach to its analysis has to be considered carefully.

Conclusion

We have presented two examples of the routes through which nurses come to engage with research. Although these are both less than conventional, they are by no means unusual in this respect, as other instances demonstrate (see for example, case studies described in Freshwater and Bishop, 2004, Chapter 7). Each individual treads a unique pathway, starting with their own attributes and preferences and encountering influences from their education, professional socialization, life experiences and sheer chance. These combine together to produce the person's attitude to all aspects of their engagement with research, including the way that they regard the processes of data analysis and interpretation.

Understanding one's intellectual heritage and valuing diverse perspectives

The diversity of nurse researchers produced by this means provides a rich resource for the profession; one that perhaps we do not sufficiently value. In our opinion, it is important for the individual to recognize the impact of their intellectual inheritance on their relationship with data, and for the research community to seek to understand the varied entities within it. We have both benefited from working together over the last ten years during which we have developed an understanding and appreciation of each other's different perspective.

Patricia has shown how an initial aptitude for mathematics in an early school leaver was transformed by the opening of a door into the possibilities presented by the biosciences of the time. Davina too points to early influences; in this case subjects presented in A level Sociology which stimulated interest and the desire to know more. Her subsequent career pathway has been a continual building of expertise in this area, through which her attitude to data analysis has been progressively refined by professional experience, wide exposure to alternative perspectives in sociology and personal research. On the other hand, Patricia's career has taken her in more than one direction, resulting in an interest in method for its own sake. The impact of a scientific training has been strong throughout.

A grounding in one or other disciplines such as these, provides an entrée to an academic community at some level. As an insider in that community, one is provided with the tools through which certain kinds of data can be analysed and discussed. However, becoming a practitioner opens other windows on to the meaning of the data that enable the analyst to serve as bridge between the worlds of research and practice.

The value of discipline-specific education

As we have seen earlier, some authorities consider that the academic discipline of nursing should be the exclusive means of preparation for nursing research. Clearly, undergraduate programmes in nursing provide the essential foundations for practice, but, by virtue of their wide scope, they can do no more than provide an introduction to a range of underlying disciplines. This is considered to be sufficient to inform the study of nursing practice, but creates a difficulty when a nursing research topic requires deeper immersion in one of the social, mathematical or biomedical sciences. In this case, we would argue, the research cannot be analysed and interpreted to a high standard unless the nurse researchers themselves have a complete preparation in that discipline. Of course, collaborative working is often successfully employed as a compromise solution, involving team members with specific expertise, but that essential bridge is difficult to create unless the nurse analyst has equal strengths in nursing and the underlying subject, and can engage on equal terms with the academic community within that area.

We do not intend to imply that this is necessary in all areas of nursing research, particularly where the work is solely based on a nursing theoretical framework. But where the research depends on the methods, techniques and theories of other disciplines, then its quality depends on the research producer acting as a professional within those disciplines. (After all, we would be very concerned if physicists were carrying out patient assessments, or sociologists delivering babies.)

The opportunities to acquire a discipline specific education in addition to nursing are relatively few and may be regarded as something of a luxury. As they so often do, nurses have seen the need to gain deeper knowledge and have taken it upon themselves to enhance their skills, using their own time and resources to great effect. But maybe we need to recognize that the addition of these skills is not a luxury for the privileged few or those who are prepared to make sacrifices, but a necessity for the establishment of the profession's secure research base.

References

Allen, D. (2001) 'Narrating nursing jurisdiction: atrocity stories and boundary-work', *Symbolic Interaction*, 24, 1–28.
—— (2004) 'Ethnomethodological insights into insider-outsider relationships in nursing ethnographies of healthcare settings', *Nursing Inquiry*, 11, 14–24.
Blaxter, L., Hughes, C. and Tight, M. (2001) *How to Research*, Buckingham: Open University Press.
Bosk, C. (1979) *Forgive and Remember: Managing Medical Failure*, Chicago, IL: University of Chicago Press.
Browne, N., Grocutt, P., Cowley, S., Cameron, J., Dealey, C., Keogh, A., Lovatt, A., Vowden, K. and Vowden, P. (2003) 'Wound care research for appropriate products (WRAP): validation of the TELER method involving users', *International Journal of Nursing Studies*, 41, 559–71.
Dingwall, R. (1977) *The Social Organisation of Health Visitor Training*, London: Croom Helm.
Douglas, J. (1967) *The Social Meanings of Suicide*, Princeton, NJ: Princeton University Press.
Durkheim, E. (1952) *Suicide (1897)*, London: Routledge and Kegan Paul.
Fairhurst, E. (1971) 'On being a patient in an orthopaedic ward: some thoughts on the definition of the situation', in A. Davis and B. Horobin (eds) *Medical Encounters: The Experience of Illness and Treatment*. London: Croom Helm.
Freshwater, D. and Bishop, V. (2004) *Nursing Research in Context: Appreciation, Application and Professional Development*, Basingstoke: Palgrave Macmillan.

Giddens, A. (1977) 'A theory of suicide', in A. Giddens (ed.) *Studies in Social and Political Theory,* London: Hutchinson.

Gilbert, N.G. and Mulkay, M. (1984) *Opening Pandora's Box: A Sociological Analysis of Scientists' Discourse*, Cambridge: Cambridge University Press.

Hughes, D. and Allen, D. (1993a) *Expanded Nursing Roles: Junior Doctors' Hours and the Hospital Division of Labour: Report for South East Thames Regional Health Authority*, Nottingham: University of Nottingham.

—— (1993b) *Inside the Black Box: Obstacles to Change in the Modern Hospital.* Nottingham: Kings Fund and Milbank Memorial Fund, Joint Health Policy Review, University of Nottingham.

Ivetic, O. and Lyne, P.A. (1990) 'Fungating and ulcerating malignant lesions: a review of the literature concerning their nature, incidence, treatment and care with discussion of the implications for nursing practice of the current state of knowledge in this field', *Journal of Advanced Nursing*, 15, 83–8.

Krebs, H.A. (1981) *Reminiscences and Reflections*, Oxford, Oxford University Press.

Krebs, H.A., Salvin, E. and Johnson, W.A. (1938) 'The formation of citric and ketoglutaric acids in the mammalian body', *Biochemical Journal*, 32, 113.

Lyne, P.A. (1994) 'The importance of measurement', *Nurse Researcher*, 1, 13–25.

Selvin, H. (1965) 'Durkheim's "Suicide": Further thoughts on a methodological classic', in R. Nisbet (ed.) *Emile Durkheim*, Englewood Cliffs, NJ: Prentice-Hall.

Strauss, A., Schatzman, L., Bucher, R., Ehrlich, D. and Sabshin, M. (1963) 'The hospital and it's negotiated order', in E. Freidson (ed.) *The Hospital in Modern Society*, New York: Free Press.

Zerubavel, E. (1979) *Patterns of Time in Hospital Life*, Chicago, IL: Chicago University Press.

Chapter 12

Relationship with multidisciplinary research teams

Sally Rees and Sue Bale

Introduction

In this chapter we present two research projects in which nurses were involved in very different capacities as part of the multidisciplinary research team: one as a novice research assistant involved in a qualitative study in an education context, and the other as an experienced researcher coordinating a clinical trial in a practice setting. The contrasts presented by these two cases illuminate some of the challenges that face nurses when working with researchers from a variety of other disciplines. We examine some of the tensions that can develop when, for example, language is used differently or misunderstandings arise about roles and responsibilities, and consider how these might be prevented or resolved. We particularly highlight the need for each professional to recognize the viewpoint and perspective of the other, thus gaining a common understanding. In our case studies we describe how this was achieved.

The terms 'multidisciplinary' 'multiprofessional' and 'interprofessional' are used to describe teams working together in health care for many purposes including research. Several authors comment on the complexity of defining these terms and also note that they are commonly used interchangeably, both within and outside the academic world (Rawson, 1994; Leathard, 1994; Scholes and Vaughan, 2002). Whilst we acknowledge this discussion, it is outside the scope of this chapter, where we adopt the term multidisciplinary. One of the key aspects of multidisciplinary team (MDT) working is collaboration. Gelling and Chatfield (2001) argue that the benefits of effective collaboration in MDTs include better-equipped researchers, increased interprofessional cohesiveness, maximum research productivity and more effective use of personnel. Working collaboratively is central to the successful completion of research projects that require the input of different professionals. National policy supports collaborative working (Department of Health, 2000; Department of Health, 2001) where nurses are recognized as having a valuable contribution to make (Department of Health, 1999). Our two case studies illustrate some of the practical realities and issues nurses need to take into account in making this contribution.

> **Case study 1: The nurse as a junior partner – Sally**
>
> The research project: *Learning to Share: The Potential for Shared Learning between Social Workers and Nurses on Qualifying Programmes in Wales* (Connor, 1995) was commissioned by the Central Council for Education and Training of Social Workers,

Cymru (CCETSW, Cymru). It was undertaken at the Cardiff Institute of Higher Education (CIHE) and led by a social work senior lecturer. The aim of the project was to explore opportunities for shared learning between social work and nurse education on qualifying programmes in Wales. The remit was to examine five issues: social work and nurse lecturers' general views about shared learning between their students; the stage at which it should take place; the programme areas believed to be the most suitable; the potential for shared placements and issues concerning the implementation of shared learning. The research comprised a curriculum analysis to establish potential areas which might be shared, followed by interviews with providers of social work and nurse education in the 13 colleges delivering qualifying courses throughout Wales ($n = 44$).

Funds were available to employ an assistant researcher. I had been working as a nurse teacher for six years, during which time there had been many changes in nurse education. When I began, nursing was taught entirely within the National Health Service (NHS) and I was employed by a Health Authority, in a hospital School of Nursing. In 1991 nurse education in Wales moved into higher education and the School went through a major transition period, finally (in 1995) becoming incorporated into the University of Wales College of Medicine (UWCM), a prestigious university with a dominant research culture and a high ranking in the 1992 Research Assessment Exercise (RAE). Alongside this move, educational requirements for nurse teachers were reviewed and all teachers were required to attain graduate status.

The assistant researcher position was advertised in the autumn of 1994 as a secondment for a nurse teacher for two days per week for three months from January to March 1995, and this is where I came in. I was appointed to this position. Until this time my research involvement had mainly been as a utilizer of published research. I had been secretary of a nursing research interest group for many years, which was interested in reviewing current evidence that could be applied to practice. A typical meeting would entail discussion of an area of research e.g. a chapter of the popular Walsh and Ford (1998) text, and how this could be implemented in practice. These meetings 'fired up' those who attended (including me) and generated enthusiasm for research and its benefits to patient care. I had not actually undertaken any research to this date and was keen to develop some research skills. This post gave me the opportunity and was especially good timing as I had just started studying for a master's degree in research methodology. The main purpose of my role was to interview all nurse educationalists using an agreed interview schedule. My knowledge and expertise of pre-registration education was therefore needed to inform the project.

Although the work was initiated and funded by the social work professional body, collaboration was sought with nurse education early on through the Welsh National Board (WNB), which at the time had responsibility *inter alia* for nurse education. Collaboration at this level was important for both the project approval and for implementing findings should the recommendations of the project require action. Following initial discussions between the two bodies, a Steering Group was set up to oversee the project, consisting of eight members representative of management, education and practice in the two professions. The Steering Group met monthly and was a valuable resource to the project and to me in my role as a novice researcher. For example, after the lead researcher and I had designed the interview schedule we took it to the Steering Group for approval. Members made very constructive comments and minor changes were made to the schedule. They were also very positive about our efforts and my involvement in the project. This affirmed to me that I was on the right track, and gave me the confidence to throw myself wholeheartedly into the work, feeling secure that I had the support of the Steering Group and could seek advice and guidance. The Steering Group was also very helpful at this stage in providing information on contacts for arranging initial interviews, and later helped to clarify issues regarding the different educational programmes. Meetings were always lively, constructive and stimulating and helped to move the research process forward in the most encouraging way for the researchers.

Although happy and excited about this opportunity, I was aware of several pressures, some of which arose from the limited time available for my part of the project. Twenty-six days (over a three-month period) were allocated for data collection. It was expected that during this short time I would also get to grips with the concepts of shared learning, familiarize myself with the necessary programmes of pre-registration education, and undertake and transcribe the interviews. I needed to 'hit the ground running'. In my first week I started making appointments to interview the 23 nurse educationalists, from departments of nursing throughout Wales. Shortly after this I started data generation. It was against this background that the research began, and a priority was to establish, with the lead researcher a common understanding of each other's professions and qualifying programmes so that we could undertake the research interviews.

Understanding each other's profession and professional world

The recognition of the need for a nurse and a social work educationalist to work together was clear in my appointment. However, it was surprising how little we knew about each other's professional worlds. I had assumed that because I had worked with social workers I automatically understood their role. This turned out not to be the case, as what I did know was only from a nurse's point of view. I knew nothing about their training. Similarly, my fellow researcher knew little about the regulation and training of nurses. There was a real need for us to spend time together just to share knowledge and develop mutual understanding. Although little dedicated time was built in for getting to know one another, there were some occasions during the project that were particularly valuable for building rapport and gaining insight into each other's professional worlds.

The first and probably most important of these, which occurred in the December of 1994, prior to the official start of the project, was when we worked together on the curriculum analysis. This work was undertaken in addition to the time allocated for this project. We spent a day at the lead researcher's house away from the phone and the hustle and bustle of work, and spread before us the different curricula documents, supplied by the participating departments of nursing and social work education. This time was an excellent grounding, providing us with the chance to discuss the complexities of each other's courses. There were, however, problems with the consistency of the material available. Some schools had sent the whole curriculum, whilst others had supplied prospectuses, course information or course handbooks. Nursing documentation was relatively sparse. This was thought to be due to the particular political climate in the early 1990s (described in Chapter 2), where a market ethos had been brought into nurse education and competition had been introduced between nursing colleges for the first time (Department of Health, 1989).

Although a true curriculum analysis had to be abandoned, this time proved to be essential in beginning to map the pre-registration nursing and social work curricula against each other; in clarifying concepts and language used in the two professions and exploring issues related to theory, practice and culture. Nursing curricula reflected Project 2000 guidance that recommended the inclusion of several academic disciplines related to nursing in the curriculum (see Bernstein, 1977) whereas social work curricula reflected a more integrated approach. There were subtle differences between the routes that allow nurses and social workers to practise in particular areas (such as child care and learning disabilities) once qualified. Placements in social work and nurse education obviously differed but there were commonalities in the support systems for learners in practice. Potential cultural differences between nursing students and social work students resulted from differences in entry criteria. Nursing students can commence training at age 17½, producing relatively young cohorts of students, whereas until recently social work students had to be over the age of 21 and are often considerably more mature than this. Exploring these issues provided an unusual opportunity to gain detailed understanding of our respective professions.

Another important time, which strengthened the professional relationship (and our personal friendship), was a joint data collection trip to North Wales in early March, which we planned together in order to conserve resources. This gave us a good opportunity to talk to each other during the car journey about developments in the project and was helpful in gaining insight into the interviews each had undertaken and themes arising from the data collected to date. With hindsight I can see the value of making opportunities for interaction between members of the MDT an integral part of the research process, rather than this being left to chance.

Developing a shared language

At a very early stage we became aware of the need to clarify some of the core concepts of the project, for example, the phrase 'joint training' had been used in the terms of reference, but we found that there was some confusion as to whether this meant joint qualification. This was probably because some joint qualifying programmes had recently been developed for nursing and social work in the field of learning disability (Evans and McCray, 1994). It was apparent that, in the same way that assumptions had been made about our understanding of each other's profession, we had also assumed a common understanding of the concepts and terms that were being used. It was imperative that there was agreement on what shared learning meant in our research. Finding clear definitions was challenging as the following extract from the report illustrates:

> A review of the literature regarding joint initiatives revealed that many authors had not attempted to clarify the terms used. Tope (1994) in her literature search noted that various terms were used interchangeably to describe interdisciplinary learning, both within and between publications. This may be due to the potentially complex nature of defining the concepts involved and the lack of agreement as to which terms should be used.
>
> (Connor, 1995, p.11)

It was important to distinguish our concept of students learning together from joint training to make clear that we were exploring opportunities for students to share some learning experiences whilst following courses leading to separate qualifications. So the term 'shared learning' was subsequently used in the interview schedule and the write up of the report. For the purpose of the study, this was defined as any learning experience that takes place between two or more professions, requiring some interaction between different professional students rather than simply being in the same place. We were surprised by the amount of effort needed to arrive at this shared articulation of the project focus, but consider that it was most important to reach this point.

Understanding the purpose of research activity for each other's profession

One of the interesting insights gained whilst working together was the different emphasis that each profession placed on the purpose and value of research. As discussed in Chapter 2 many discourses influence the impetus, funding and implementation of research, and this was evident in our project. For both of us there were managerial and professional discourses at play but these were different for each researcher. For the social work education department and the professional body the main impetus for exploring the possibilities for shared learning was very practical: it was seen as a precursor to a future project where shared learning could be piloted in practice. The department was in a former polytechnic and was not, at that time, under pressure to participate in the RAE. However, for the School of Nursing and the WNB, involvement in research was important in its own right, because of the formal links with the research-led College of Medicine and its RAE driven research culture. There was a strengthening emphasis on the need to publish research findings in reputable nursing journals and to disseminate studies at nursing conferences. It was also important to me personally to gain as many research skills and as much experience as I could from the secondment. Once I had made these objectives clear to the lead researcher she provided development opportunities for me during the project.

The purpose of the particular research for each of the members of the research team is likely to influence the direction of future collaboration, and thus it is important that these are understood at an early stage, so that the implication of the findings for future work may be anticipated. This research project uncovered several barriers that would need to be overcome in order for shared learning to take place. The potential for practical development was therefore found to be limited under current circumstances. However, it also revealed the potential for shared learning between occupational therapy and social work. Consequently, the follow up pilot project led by the social work educationalists involved collaboration between these two professions (Connor, 1998) and the formal participation of nursing ceased. However, since I had shared my personal aspirations to develop my research skills with the lead researcher, I was given the opportunity to continue my involvement after the official three-month period, on an informal basis in my own time. This enabled me to take part in some of the data analysis and a little of the report writing under the lead researcher's guidance, giving me a sense of great personal satisfaction. Differences in the professional discourses to which we were subject continued to affect the way we treated the outcome of the study. The lead researcher wrote up the final report for the funding body (Connor, 1995), but this was not submitted for publication and remains unpublished. However, for me, dissemination of the findings and producing a publication in a refereed journal was very important. Consequently, I pursued ways of jointly disseminating, and publishing this work. I therefore précised the report into a research article with the consent of the lead researcher and submitted it for joint publication which was accepted (Connor and Rees, 1997). When this was successfully achieved, I felt that I taken my first steps as a research producer.

Case study 2: When laboratory meets nursing: the nurse as project supervisor in wound healing research – Sue

The next case study presents a multi-centre, commercially funded investigation in which nurses managed the project, coordinating the work of other health professionals and laboratory-based scientists. At the time I was employed as Director of Nursing Research in a renowned centre of excellence in wound healing research, having had some 16 years' experience in clinical practice, research and commercial trials in that field. My role was to supervise and monitor the conduct of the work, ensuring compliance with the protocol and that the data generated were accurate, consistent, complete, and auditable to recognized standards of good practice (International Committee on Harmonisation and Good Clinical Practice, 1996). In clinical wound healing research, nurses are often the most appropriate professionals to deliver the study protocol. When this study was undertaken (1998–9), I selected one of the eight research nurses that I managed to be the project manager and lead research nurse. My role in the study included: advising on the study design, liaising with the other centres and the pharmaceutical company, defining and monitoring progress, making the ethical application, and developing and supporting the lead research nurse.

The project (Krishnamoorthy et al., 2003) was commissioned by a commercial pharmaceutical company as part of a programme of work on the development of new wound healing interventions for chronic wounds such as venous leg ulcers. One of these interventions is a living skin equivalent, skin grown from discarded foreskins of circumcised baby boys. For patients with venous leg ulceration research was needed to measure the effect of good, standard care (compression bandages only) compared to the addition of living skin equivalent. A randomized controlled trial (RCT) was indicated as the best design to answer the question of effectiveness of an intervention (Sullivan-Bolyai and Grey, 2002). The design was agreed in consultation with the participating centres and the company.

Reaching this stage of the project was quite straightforward for us as a group of experienced trialists and we were clear about the next steps. I felt confident that, with my support, the research nurse would enjoy the challenges associated with coordinating different professionals and that the project would be completed successfully within the defined time-scale, something that we had achieved many times before. Therefore my initial feelings were that this was routine work, which would be enjoyable and provide us with an opportunity to become familiar with a very new innovation in wound care.

Defining roles and responsibilities

The key research questions were as follows:

- Is living skin equivalent an effective treatment for patients with venous leg ulceration?
- Do the transplanted fibroblasts remain active?
- Is this an acceptable treatment for patients?
- Is this a practical treatment for nurses to deliver?

In order to be able to answer these questions, the expertise of several different professionals was needed in order to measure ulcer status and cellular activity, and assess patient acceptability and the implications for nursing practice. Therefore, experts from four professional backgrounds (nurse, scientist, doctor and pharmacist) were recruited. Their roles included:

- Nurses – me as project supervisor advising on the study design and overseeing the project and the lead research nurse who had delegated responsibility for ensuring that GCP standards were adhered to.
- Scientist – advising on laboratory methods and responsible for processing and analysing tissue samples.
- Doctor – monitoring patients' physical health and taking tissue samples.
- Commercial pharmacist – representing the commissioners and funders of the research, with responsibility for patient safety, monitoring GCP standards and the quality of trial outcome, as well as providing statistical and methodological support.

We felt that it was important that we understood each other's roles and responsibilities, a view shared by Henneman et al. (1995) and Gelling and Chatfield (2001). The scientist, doctor and commercial pharmacist each had discrete and clearly defined responsibilities. Once the study design was agreed, each had a function to perform that was largely independent of the others. They spent a fixed amount of time working in the unit and did not form part of the permanent research team, unlike the nurses. The philosophy of the unit, as developed by the management team, was one of multidisciplinary team working where no one professional group took precedence. Here, participation in a project was based upon an individual's skills and abilities to get the job done.

The team met together on two occasions during the initial stages of the work and agreed that the trial should include four arms: control with compression alone and compression plus three different frequencies of application of living skin equivalent. An independent statistician calculated the sample size required. Consensus was also achieved for the study outcomes, which comprised: time to healing and percentage reduction in ulcer area; cellular activity, determined by the survival and functions of the transplanted fibroblasts and patient satisfaction. However, one issue caused considerable debate within the team: it could not reach consensus on the frequency of measuring and monitoring cellular activity. To get the most meaningful results the scientist required weekly ulcer bed punch biopsy measuring 10–20 mm in diameter. This would enable tracking of cellular survival and activity over time, ultimately providing optimal intervals for application of the living skin equivalent. In order to obtain the best data the scientist required up to 13 tissue samples of this quantity of tissue for every patient. The nurse, doctor and commercial pharmacist were of the opinion that it would be unethical as well as impractical to ask patients to donate this amount of tissue this frequently, as it is often an uncomfortable procedure. All team members appreciated that it would also be unethical to conduct a study where the data would not be meaningful. This was the first tension in the multi-professional team, where we needed to understand each other's perspective.

Understanding team members' priorities

The scientist was understandably concerned and frustrated at the prospect of not being able to provide a high standard of science. Clinical staff were concerned for the well-being of the participants. There was the potential here for a breakdown in the smooth running of the project, if this difference in priorities could not be resolved.

In order to improve the scientist's understanding of the process for the patient of donating tissue, the doctor and myself invited him to a clinic where tissue biopsies were being harvested. Here, he could appreciate the detailed explanation required of the nurse in securing informed consent, the skill of the doctor in harvesting the tissue, and of course the great inconvenience to the patient donating the tissue. On the other hand, he was able to explain to the other members of the research team the scientific consideration of wanting to obtain the best data possible. By bringing all parties together each could appreciate the perspective of the other and ethical, scientific and practical considerations discussed, resulting in an acceptable compromise. An agreement was made to collect tissue biopsies once a month throughout the study, so that a maximum of five biopsies would be required. This would provide the scientist with sufficient frequency of tissue samples to track cellular activity through the study period, whilst minimizing invasive procedures for the patient. Previous experience in undertaking studies where patients were asked to donate tissue samples led myself and the doctor to conclude that monthly sampling was likely to be an acceptable frequency for patients. One of the key factors in achieving this outcome was effective communication, which Gelling and Chatfield (2001) highlight as one of the most important elements of a successful collaborative partnership.

Mentoring and supporting the research manager

During my career I have acted as project supervisor for numerous projects involving multidisciplinary teams and have an awareness of both the practicalities to be considered and the way these are viewed or prioritized by team members. On this occasion, my role was to support, mentor and develop the research nurse as project manager and to share this experience. Clearly, for this study, it was important for her to consider: patients' availability and commitments; doctors' work schedules and availability; the time and equipment required by the scientist at the time of tissue harvesting and for subsequent sample processing; the availability of a suitable clinical environment to conduct the research (i.e. research clinic or patient's home) and availability, storage and delivery of the living skin equivalent, bandages and other supplies.

Once we had charted these elements we had to consider the contribution and requirements of each team member and the patients, to ensure that treatments were given and data collected according to the protocol. We called a meeting where the practicalities of the project were discussed and each member of the team had an opportunity to describe their role and what they required in order to ensure success.

The project manager was responsible for ensuring that the project ran smoothly and all team members fulfilled their commitments and worked together. At the outset of the study, she was concerned that medical and scientific colleagues would resent the authority vested in her role and that this would lead to tensions within the team, possibly adversely affecting the success of the project. As described in Part 1, medical discourses cast nurses in a subordinate position relative to doctors rather than equal partners. This concern has been shared by others (Porter, 1991, 1995, 1996), where conflict between nurses and doctors is described in conjunction with the ways in which doctors exert power over nurses. Coombs (Coombs, 2004) suggests that it is traditional, in the decision-making process, for nurses to perceive doctors to be domineering, and that doctors perceive nurses to be weak and unprepared to take responsibility. However, successful working relationships have been reported in an intensive care setting (Coombs, 2003, 2004), a specialist area where nurses have developed expertise which is acknowledged by their medical colleagues. A similar situation obtains in wound healing.

My role was to support the lead research nurse and encourage her to identify, anticipate and plan for problems that could affect the progress of the project. Some of this knowledge she already had and I supplemented this by drawing on my past experience and talking things through with her. I was able to reassure her that, in the event of interprofessional tensions arising, the management team would be supportive of her in this role and that I could intervene if this were necessary.

The co-ordination of a complex study such as this was a major challenge for the lead research nurse. With so many different elements there would be many situations where the study protocol could be violated. Patients were referred from district and practice nurses, GPs, and clinic staff. They visited the study centre to receive explanations before giving consent. This was a high priority for the team on account of the invasive procedures involved (donating tissue biopsies). Once enrolled, the first visit was arranged by the nurse, ensuring that this was convenient for the patient, that the doctor was available to harvest the tissue biopsy and also that the timing was right to allow the scientist to process it. However, as the study began and patients were recruited, logistical problems were encountered. Owing to other work commitments, the doctor and scientist were sometimes unable to attend the research clinic for planned patient visits, and it took time for the research nurses to locate them. This caused inconvenience to the patient, wasted nursing time and generated the potential for conflict. This tension was later defused when the lead research nurse held a debriefing, where each was able to discuss their issues and understand the other's perspective.

My previous experience as project supervisor gave me confidence to act in support of the lead research nurse in planning and coordinating the work and dealing with potential interprofessional conflict. In clinical practice it is historically unusual for a nurse to take a key role in patient care. Coombs (2004) highlights many situations where medical staff made clinical decisions about patient care without reference to nurses delivering care. In addition, she draws attention to tension and conflict that results when nurses feel intimidated by doctors and do not raise their clinical concerns. In this project, it was essential that these concerns were raised and successfully resolved.

Discussion

Our case studies have highlighted the diverse external factors that impact upon MDT research. They illustrate that MDT research does not take place in a vacuum but is influenced by the historical, social and political context in which it takes place. The case studies have identified a number of occasions where there was the potential for conflict. The influence of some of these factors and the professional discourse regarding their genesis and resolution will be considered, identifying some practical lessons arising from our experiences.

Developing shared understanding

The need for planned time embedded in the research to allow for exploration of each others' perspectives on the research to be undertaken, and for developing understanding of each others' viewpoints, cannot be underestimated. In Sally's study the opportunity to gain insight into each other's professional worlds of practice and culture could so easily have been missed having a direct impact on the quality of the research.

Nurses and social workers share a similar professional history and both have an educational pathway progressing from vocational training into higher education. So in this respect there was likely to be equal status and limited potential for conflict overall between them when working in MDTs. This was certainly Sally's experience. In addition, her project concerned only two people and two professional groups and sharing of information as professional colleagues was required for the project success. However, even in this situation, considerable effort had to be expended to ensure the use of a common language and to remedy hitherto unsuspected gaps in inter-professional understanding. On the other hand, scientists, doctors and nurses take different pathways to higher education and the evolutionary histories of their professions differ markedly. Sue's project involved a much larger and more diverse team, including at least seven people and four professional groups, some of whom were already working together while others joined the team for the project. This added layers of complexity with more potential for misunderstandings and conflicts. However, it was essential that, as patients were participating in this research, the research ran smoothly and that conflict was not allowed to develop to such an extent that it interfered with the project. Again, opportunities to increase understanding of colleagues' roles and priorities were created, although not formally planned. The evident impact of such activities on project success suggests the importance, in multidisciplinary research, of formally planning them into the timetable.

The need for good management

We have also illustrated the importance of good management for multidisciplinary research. In Sally's study, the Steering Group, and in Sue's study, the management team, were instrumental in negotiating the researchers through the research process. In both studies the experience of this management was very positive. The groups were well organized and the group members were highly committed to the aims of the research. This kind of support is not only desirable but also essential if true understanding and collaboration is to be achieved.

Understanding the political context

Both cases demonstrate the impact of the political context in shaping the research conducted by practice-based professions. Sally's project was initiated in response to current developments in multidisciplinary practice. The major legislative changes in the Children Act (1989) and the NHS and Community Care Act (1990) had emphasized the importance of professional collaboration to the delivery of quality services and had brought social worker and nursing professional responsibilities closer together in order to provide 'seamless care'. Professional bodies echoed this requirement (UKCC, 1992; Central Council for Education and Training of Social Work, 1995). The underlying premise was that learning together would enhance practice. However, the smooth running of the project was impeded by other events in the political agenda in nurse education. For example, the newly introduced market philosophy made it difficult to obtain curricula from many colleges of nursing. Government guidance regarding Project 2000 with the drive towards separating the subjects to be taught in nursing militated against sharing with the integrated curricula of social work education.

In contrast, Sue's project was shaped by a set of forces that included the politics of higher education and a strong commercial imperative. The research unit was largely self-sustaining, with experience of successful commercially funded projects and in preparing for the 2001 RAE, the generation of external funding was prioritized in the university's research strategy. Linking with commercial organizations was perceived as one way to respond to these pressures and, at the same time, allow the conduct of research with new technologies for the benefit of patient care.

The role of the nurse researcher in MDTs

These case studies demonstrate some of the varied ways in which nurses engage with and contribute to research. Our examples span the breadth of the research continuum explored in Chapter 5. Sally was looking for an opportunity for professional growth alongside her teaching role as a part-time activity. Already a utilizer of research, she became a 'novice research producer'. The secondment gave her experience in interviewing, transcribing and data analysis. She also gained the opportunity to develop writing and presentation skills. From this foundation Sally was able to use her enhanced knowledge of the research process to inform her teaching role, and to continue her development as a research producer (Rees, 1998). Sue, as Director of Nursing Research in the Unit, was a full-time, experienced researcher and an expert in her particular field. As producer, her work demonstrated high-level characteristics, with membership of international committees, a track record of gaining funding and participation in multi-site and MDT research. However, in the present project her role was complex. She was supervisor of the research and was also concerned with developing the project manager and supporting her in the management of the research nurses and other members of the MDT. In this role Sue was influential in the growth and development of several other research nurses' knowledge and skills.

Conclusion

The whole concept of research multidisciplinarity has moved much higher up the agenda in health and higher education policy, appearing as a quality criterion in the 2001 RAE. This raises the question of the role of nurses in the teams which are established to carry out this model of research activity. We concur with Lorentzon (1998), who argues that a dual approach is needed, where nurses contribute to the research process both in a uni-disciplinary capacity and as part of a multidisciplinary research team. She believes that this will allow the uniqueness of nursing research to continue, whilst developing a collegial, collaborative approach that strengthens an emerging trend towards equality of status with multidisciplinary research.

References

Bernstein, B. (1977) *Class, Codes and Control: Towards a Theory of Educational Transmission*, London: Routledge and Kegan Paul.

Central Council for Education and Training of Social Work (1995) *Rules and Requirements for the Diploma in Social Work*, revised edn, London: Central Council for Education and Training of Social Work.

Connor, C. (1995) *Learning to Share: The Potential for Shared Learning between Social Workers and Nurses on Qualifying Programmes in Wales*, Cardiff: Central Council for Education and Training of Social Work, Wales.

—— (1998) *A Problem Shared: An Evaluation of Shared Learning Between Social Work and Occupational Therapy Students on Qualifying Programmes*, Cardiff: University of Wales Institute Cardiff, University of Wales College of Medicine.

Connor, C. and Rees, S. (1997) 'Ways Forward for shared learning between nursing and social work students', *Nurse Education Today*, 17(6), 494–501.

Coombs, M. (2003) 'Power and conflict in intensive care clinical decision making', *Intensive and Critical Care Nursing*, 19, 125–35.

—— (2004) *Power and Conflict Between Doctors and Nurses: Breaking Through the Inner Circle in Clinical Care*, London: Routledge.

Department of Health (1989) *Working for Patients. Education and Training. Working Paper 10*, London: Department of Health.

—— (1999) *Making a Difference: Strengthening the Nursing, Midwifery and Health Visiting Contribution to Health and Healthcare*, London: Department of Health.

—— (2000) *The NHS Plan: A Plan for Investment, a Plan for Reform*, London: Department of Health.

—— (2001) *Shifting the Balance of Power: The Next Step*, London: Department of Health.

Evans, N. and McCray, J. (1994) *Diploma in Social Work/Registered Nurse Mental Handicap Joint Training: The Portsmouth Experience*, London: ENB/CCETSW.

Gelling, L. and Chatfield, D. (2001) 'Research collaboration', *Nurse Researcher*, 9, 4–16.

Henneman, E.A., Lee, J.L. and Cohen, J.I. (1995) 'Collaboration: a concept analysis', *Journal of Advanced Nursing*, 21, 103–9.

International Committee on Harmonisation and Good Clinical Practice (1996) *Guideline for Good Practice* (ICH Harmonised Tripartite Guideline).

Krishnamoorthy, L., Harding, K., Griffiths, D., Moore, K., Leaper, D., Poskitt, K., Sibbald, R.G., Brassard, A., Dolynchuk, K., Adams, J. and Whyman, M. (2003) 'The clinical and histological effects of Dermagraft in the healing of chronic venous leg ulcers', *Phlebology*, 18, 12–22.

Leathard, A. (1994) 'Inter-professional developments in Britain: An overview', in A. Leathard (ed.) *Going Inter-Professional: Working Together for Health and Social Welfare*, London: Routledge.

Lorentzon, M. (1998) 'The way forward: nursing research or collaborative health care research?', *Journal of Advanced Nursing*, 27, 675–6.

Porter, S. (1991) 'A participant observational study of power relationships between doctors and nurses in a general hospital', *Journal of Advanced Nursing*, 16, 728–35.

—— (1995) *Nursing's Relationship with Medicine*, Aldershot: Avebury.

—— (1996) 'Contra-Foucault: nurses, soldiers and power', *Sociology*, 30, 59–78.

Rawson, D. (1994) 'Models of interprofessional work: Likely theories and possibilities', in A. Leathard (Ed.) *Going Interprofessional: Working Together for Health and Social Welfare*, London: Routledge.

Rees, S. (1998) '"Going into Blue": An Exploration of Newly Qualified Nurse Experience and Perceptions of the Staff Nurse Role', Cardiff: University of Wales, School of Social Administration.

Scholes, J. and Vaughan, B. (2002) 'Cross-boundary working: implications for the multiprofessional team', *Journal of Clinical Nursing*, 11, 399–408.

Sullivan-Bolyai, S. and Grey, M. (2002) 'Experimental and quasi-experimental designs', in G. Lobiondo-Wood and J. Haber (eds) *Nursing Research: Methods, Critical Appraisal and Utilization*, St Louis, MO: Mosby.

UKCC (1992) *Code of Professional Conduct*, London: UKCC.

Walsh, M. and Ford, P. (1998) *Nursing Rituals: Research and Rational Actions*, Oxford: Heinemann Nursing.

Chapter 13

Disseminating your research findings

Philip Satherley and Patricia Lyne

Introduction

In this chapter our focus is on the dissemination of research findings and the way that the past and current environment of nursing research has affected the relationship between research and practice as mediated by the process of dissemination. In introducing the chapter we will first describe the 'typical' dissemination chain, i.e. the series of processes through which research outputs find their way to the hands (or computer screens) of those who read and use them. Along the way there are factors which affect the rate and direction of progress. We will argue that there are particular circumstances which impact on this process and that these can have an adverse effect on the incremental development of the kind of body of knowledge that characterizes the more mature research disciplines. The case studies which follow emphasize what we have learnt about the importance of developing a planned rather than reactive dissemination strategy. In case studies 1 and 2 we will draw out lessons for potential authors and discuss the relationship between author, the review process and the written output. Case study 3 will examine the way in which published findings are interpreted and used to inform practice.

The dissemination process

Lomas and Haynes (1987) describe dissemination as 'the spread of knowledge from its source to health care practitioners'. This very wide definition encompasses all means, informal as well as formal, whereby research can inform practice communities. Whilst acknowledging the importance of other avenues for dissemination, such as conferences, guidelines, information leaflets (Blackburn *et al.*, 1997) and workshops, we will confine our attention in this chapter to publications via peer-reviewed printed or electronic journals.

Dissemination of research findings is an essential constituent of, and closely coupled to, evidence-based health care; a system whose other components include ensuring practitioners have the intellectual and practical means to assess evidence (Lyne *et al.*, 2002), and translation of knowledge into practice (van Weel, 2003). It is the process through which research findings are placed in the public arena and then become the raw material for the evidence industry. However, research outputs play other important roles in the varied communities to which they are directed, including academia, education and management as well as practice (see Chapter 5 for further discussion). The issues discussed in this chapter need to be viewed in the light of the intended audience for, and purpose of, dissemination activities.

The dissemination chain following the production of a finished paper involves the selection of the target journal, the review process, the editorial response to the submitted work, publication and the interpretation of the work by the readership. The final outcome is influenced by events occurring at all stages of this process, as our case studies will illustrate.

Selection of the journal

Nursing-related research is one of the fastest growing fields of health care research (Rafferty *et al.*, 2000). The volume of printed outputs has increased considerably over the past ten years, with over 800 active nursing journals listed in Ulrich's Periodicals Directory (sourced May 2005). Work of relevance to nursing also appears in a range of other publications.

Regularly published printed sources have a long history, with the first recorded medical journal *Medica Curiosa* being produced in 1684. The establishment of a journal by its founding authors can play an important part in the history of a profession and reflects an intellectual or practical response to a current situation. For example, the founder of *The Lancet*, Dr Thomas Wakley, took a stand against existing medical dogma.

> Indeed, we trust that mystery and ignorance will shortly be considered synonymous. Ceremonies, and signs, have now lost their charms; hieroglyphics, and gilded serpents, their power to deceive.
>
> (Wakley, 1823, p. 1)

This philosophy helped lay the foundations for the evidence-based movement, initiating a relationship between the production of up-to-date research for journals and their readership.

During the lifetime of a journal its underlying philosophy evolves in response to events in the professional and academic environments. The emergence of new journals mirrors developments in professional thinking and indeed the emergence of new disciplines or sub-disciplines that have different expectations about the communication of knowledge. The more specialized the research discipline, the more uniform these expectations and norms (Waddell, 2002). In contrast, the outputs of nursing research cross many professional boundaries and have to satisfy a broad spectrum of expectations, including an academic need for scholarly achievement and an equal need to inform practice.

Selection of the target journal for a paper has to be informed by consideration of many aspects of the available outlets. Its subsequent progress will be affected by the degree to which the paper meets the requirements of the journal to which it is submitted. On receipt of the paper the editor will decide if the paper is suitable and recommend its further progress to peer review. The papers produced by nurses, reflecting the research that is of significance to the professions, are often of a 'non standard' nature, i.e. they do not fit easily into well-recognized dissemination routes or conform to long established criteria in the parent disciplines. It can, therefore, be difficult to predict whether a particular journal will accept a 'non traditional' paper and to convince editors and reviewers of the merits of work which falls outside certain very firmly held ways of thinking. Our first case study is an example of this process.

The review process and editorial response

The next crucial step in the chain is the reaction of the reviewer(s) to the paper, as expressed in their comments to the author and advice to the editor. This can be a disheartening phase of the dissemination process, especially to the neophyte author. Reviewer's comments typically take one of four forms:

1   Acceptance of the paper as it stands (a very rare occurrence) or subject to minor amendments (such as including additional references or tightening up some conclusions).
2   Acceptance subject to substantial revision (this indicates that the paper shows potential but needs considerable further work – journals vary in the extent to which they specify exactly what is required).
3   Rejection with possible submission in revised form. (The reviewers are unsure whether the paper can reach the required standard but consider that it is worthwhile to try. There is no guarantee of acceptance after revision.)
4   Rejection with no possibility of resubmission. (The reviewers are of the opinion that the paper cannot be brought up to the required level or that it cannot be amended to fit within the scope of the journal. They may suggest an alternative outlet.)

The first of these is very good news and the last indicates that this is the end of the line as far as that particular journal is concerned, but at least the authors know where they stand. The third and fourth are often unwelcome, as they indicate that there is much additional work to be done and the authors have to decide whether the likelihood of a successful resubmission justifies the amount of effort this will take. Our personal experience leads us to believe that these two responses have a considerable impact on composition of the cohort of papers that are resubmitted to journals and thus on the body of the work that is eventually published.

The interpretation of the work by the readership

Much of the work concerning dissemination of knowledge has focused on the obstacles associated with getting research into practice, i.e. the journey from paper to bedside. These barriers are well documented, from organizational and cultural issues (NHS, 1996; Cronenwett, 1995), to information overload (Carter, 1996) and education (McDonnell et al., 1997). More recent studies have sought to bring all these strands of thought together, to develop a framework taking into account the nature of evidence being used, facilitation required and quality of context for practitioners (Rycroft-Malone et al., 2004).

The first step on this part of the dissemination route is the 'creation' of evidence through the appraisal of primary sources and the synthesis of research findings. The most highly esteemed source under the hierarchy of evidence model (Sackett et al., 1996) is the randomized control trial and subsequent systematic review of effectiveness. Organizations such as the Cochrane Collaboration produce reviews which investigate the effects of interventions and, where appropriate, evidence is pooled to provide researchers and research users with answers to clinical questions.

Research which does not adopt the clinical trial design faces a challenging route into the evidence base for practice. Non-experimental and especially qualitative research has come a long way towards being accepted by the health professions in recent years. There are journals dedicated to qualitative inquiry such as *Qualitative Health Research* and many which include similar work such as *Social Science and Medicine* and *Clinical Effectiveness in Nursing*. A key text based on work commissioned by the Health Technology Assessment Programme (Murphy *et al.*, 1998) summarized current qualitative research methods in health technology assessment. Arguments for the inclusion of such work into the evidence base have reached a sophisticated level (Lyne *et al.*, 2002; Popay *et al.*, 1998; Dixon-Woods *et al.*, 2001), with the wider medical profession beginning to recognize its potential (Banyard and Miller, 1998). The interpretative nature of qualitative outputs necessitates a certain amount of subjective interpretation by the reader. This has a considerable impact on how it can inform practice. Synthesis of qualitative studies is difficult to achieve, therefore research findings from individual projects are often left 'stranded' and fail to inform practice. Methods for the synthesis of qualitative work are currently under development (Walsh and Downe, 2005; Thorne *et al.*, 2004).

It is here that nursing research faces some particular pressures which shape its subsequent impact and growth. The outputs may be judged not only on the basis of research quality but also on their ability to become integrated into an evidence base and to be usable in practice by professionals in clinical practice, education and management. However, much research in nursing is legitimately undertaken for purposes other than the immediate production of evidence. It may be a methodological study, contributing to the nursing research repertoire of techniques or instrumentation. Alternatively, it could have a purely scholarly purpose, throwing light on important ethical, professional or theoretical concerns. Work of this nature cannot be interpreted through the lens of evidence-based health care.

Case study 1: Relationship between author and editor

Despite the attention that has been given to the development of strategies for nursing research dissemination (Scullion, 2002; Waddell, 2002), little has been written about the realities of getting a paper into press. Veronica Bishop (2004) touches on her experiences of the relationship between publisher and author, and Newell (2000) shares his experiences of working on the editorial board of *Clinical Effectiveness in Nursing*. Such accounts are rare.

The first of our case studies is not drawn from our personal experience but is based on a published account that we found to be most illuminating, as it very honestly reports the authors' attempts to have an article accepted. The authors present this as a case study to demonstrate the importance of selecting the most appropriate outlet. We provide a different emphasis by highlighting the factors of significance for the acceptance of a paper which, like so many in nursing, does not fall neatly into a recognized category.

Van Teijlingen and Hundley (2002), describe the process of attempting to publish a paper on the lessons learnt from conducting a pilot study (Van Teijlingen *et al.*, 2001). The reported work, conducted by a group of nurses and public health experts, was a series of pilot studies preparatory to a survey of maternity services in Scotland. They found that very little had been written about the importance of pilot work in this field and so, whilst the completed survey was of relevance to a particular nursing community, the methodological lessons from the pilot phase could have application to many areas of research. It was their original intention to focus on these lessons and to share their insights, because presentations on this topic had aroused considerable interest.

Whilst the impetus to publish arose because the authors felt they had something important to say, they were also conscious of needing to achieve recognition for the work and their department:

> As we were approaching the 2001 RAE [Research Assessment Exercise] our university placed considerable importance on being seen to publish in 'high impact' academic journals.
>
> (Van Teijlingen and Hundley, 2002, p. 509)

The authors were ready to submit in the summer of 1999, in the knowledge that publication could take up to 18 months and that the RAE census date for publication was 31 December 2000. They first targeted *Social Science and Medicine*, a journal of international standing with a high impact rating. Presumably the authors considered that the methodological content of their paper would be sufficiently innovative and of wide interest to satisfy the requirements of this journal. The editor was not of the same mind, replying one month after submission:

> We rarely publish 'methodological' papers, and even as a 'Research Note' this is rather slight. Also, our international readership has to be kept in mind, and this is very UK-orientated. It seems that it might be more suitable for the (UK) nursing or maternity care literature.
>
> (Van Teijlingen and Hundley, 2002, p. 509)

This was a clear message that the methodological focus was not of interest and of insufficiently wide relevance. Although disappointing, such a message is useful in that it provides the rejected author with some information that can be used in the future. The authors then turned their attention to *The Lancet*. Their decision was related to the speed of turn around of this journal. They received a rapid rejection, stating simply that the paper would be better placed elsewhere, and the same fate befell their next attempt, which was submission to the *British Medical Journal*. Once again, the response was brief and contained no detailed reasons for rejection.

These three applications had occupied almost four months and it was now early September 1999. The authors next took the decision to submit to public health journals, whose readership covered researchers and practitioners in public health and social medicine. They first turned to the *Journal of Epidemiology and Community Health*, which features a section entitled 'Theory and Methods'. It was rejected, without review, after six weeks on the grounds that:

> Due to a severe shortage of space, we need to make some difficult decisions based mainly on the suitability of the paper for an international audience and its originality. I regret to say that we are unable to accept the paper for publication.
>
> (Van Teijlingen and Hundley, 2002, p. 510)

As in the case of *Social Science and Medicine* the rejection contains hints about a lack of originality and international appeal. The authors do not tell us whether they made any changes to the paper in the light of these messages, or sent any supporting letter making the case for originality and wider relevance. This was closely followed by a submission to the *Journal of Public Health*, in mid-January 2000, with another rapid editorial rejection (two weeks) which simply stated that the paper was unsuitable for the journal. By now, eight months had passed since the initial submission, with five editorial rejections and very little in the way of editorial guidance which might help the authors become more successful. The paper had been appraised by at least five research evaluators, presumably from social science and medical backgrounds. Thus far, the effect of their appraisal had been to stall the publication of this paper.

The *Journal of Advanced Nursing* (JAN), which has a worldwide nursing audience, was the final choice for submission. The authors admit that, with hindsight, this should probably have been an earlier target, as JAN welcomes papers on methodological issues in nursing research. Its impact factor is high for a nursing journal, but lower than all the others to which the paper was previously submitted.

Almost five months after submission, the editor replied to tell the authors that the paper had been sent for review and that both referees considered it had promise, but that a major revision was required, shifting the focus from the methodological issues to the results of the pilot studies. So the paper was rewritten and finally accepted for publication on 16 January 2001. It was published, too late for the current RAE, in a section of the journal called 'Methodological issues in nursing research' which focuses on methodological innovation and lessons learnt from the utilization of existing methods.

The case study summarized here presents a fascinating example of the interplay between authors, editors, reviewers and the context in which attempts to publish take place. Our reflection on this published case led us to consider a number of issues which are relevant to the themes of this book.

The pressure to publish

The academic agenda, directed towards the 2001 RAE was a key factor in shaping the choice of target journal. The authors aimed first at high status, high impact journals. The 'impact factor' is a means of assessing the frequency with which a journal has been cited in a particular year (Amin and Mabe, 2000) and has become an acknowledged quality indicator for journals, researchers and institutions in disciplines such as the biosciences and medicine. The predominant scientific discourse accepts this convention. However, in emergent disciplines such as nursing, this is not necessarily the case and a high impact journal does not necessarily reach all the intended audience. This point was explicitly made by the panel that judged the Nursing Unit of Assessment in RAE (2001) (Bond, 2002) and has been reinforced in the emergent criteria for the operation of panels in the 2008 RAE.

The timing of their original attempt was unfortunate in that pressure on journals was at its highest. By the time they submitted the paper to JAN, it was too late for publication by the census date and pressure had diminished. There is, of course, no means of judging whether an earlier submission to JAN would have been more successful, but there is no doubt that the imperative of the RAE distorted the smooth flow of submissions to all journals and placed additional demands on authors and editors at that time. This subsequently diminished and will undoubtedly increase again before the next RAE.

Falling between many stools

The case study does not contain the original paper that the authors wished to publish, but they tell us that its focus was the lessons they had learnt in conducting pilot studies. It was clearly, then, not a standard research report or a full-scale methodological study (for example, describing the development of a new technique, or testing the properties of a measure). In the end, in order to achieve publication, the authors responded to reviewers' comments and reshaped the paper with more emphasis on the results of the pilot study, so that it became something akin to a preliminary report. One wonders whether the original message that the authors wished to convey was lost in this process.

Matching the aims and scope of the journal

In addition to their more-or-less well defined quality criteria, peer reviewed journals invariably have specific inclusion criteria. *Social Science and Medicine* for example states clearly that it is keen to publish *findings* or *reviews* which are of general interest to an *international* readership of social scientists, health practitioners and policy makers. The *Journal of Advanced Nursing* aims and scope communicate the need to inform and explore practice *worldwide*, having a sound scientific or theoretical basis reflecting the internationalism of nursing. These criteria constitute the first filter. This case study clearly shows how these were applied in two cases, at least. An obvious lesson for the aspiring author is the importance of understanding what they mean and avoiding the waste of time and effort which results when they are disregarded.

Locating the study in a body of work

We can only speculate about the content of the original paper, but it evidently did not make the case for its quality to the satisfaction of the reviewers. The version of the paper that was eventually published clearly located the study in a methodological context, stating that the full results and the associated problems with pilot studies, which then inform the major study, are rarely reported (Van Teijlingen *et al.*, 2001). The authors present data from the pilot study, together with technical, political and organizational detail concerning this work. Although this was a local study it was written up in such a way that a reader in another care system could extract information of relevance to their own situation. In this modification of their original paper the authors were able to demonstrate its wider relevance and, by locating it as part of a progressive body of work, to demonstrate a satisfactory level of quality.

Attending to the editorial comment

Editorial rejection is always disappointing. It is easier to bear if the stated reasons for rejection are clear and comprehensible, and the author is assured that the reviewers have carefully considered the paper and can give a detailed rationale for their decision, together with suggestions for improvement. Conversely, if little explanation is given, the author suffers from both disappointment and frustration that may impact on the progress of their work or their willingness to try again. In this case study the editorial comments repeatedly referred to the paper as being too UK-orientated and not suitable for an international audience. At this stage it might have been more worthwhile to either ensure that the study had relevance for a worldwide audience by grounding in an existing body of work or publishing in a more UK-centric journal.

This case study of an unusual and helpful publication brings to light several less obvious aspects of the first steps in the dissemination chain and shows how they can affect progress to publication.

Case study 2: Relationship between author and peer review process

After a paper has been accepted at editorial level it is sent to two or three external peer reviewers, usually with authors' details removed in an attempt to assure anonymity, although if the reviewers are centrally involved in the field of study they are likely to be able to make a good guess at the authorship. Each journal has a database of national and international reviewers, with proven track-records in publishing and who are considered knowledgeable in their particular field (Emden, 1996). Peer review is the accepted model for ensuring that knowledge is challenged, refined and then accepted or rejected by the scientific community (Holt *et al.*, 2000). It has been long established as an effective means for communication, being the most constructive way to enhance and develop a programme of work through critical evaluation by professional peers. It can ensure that not only is the nitty-gritty of the research addressed, but that the paper communicates *elegantly* to the reader. The following case study describes the peer review process through which a paper ('Narrating Nursing Jurisdiction: "Atrocity Stories" and Boundary-Work') was accepted for publication by *Symbolic Interaction*

(Allen, 2001). This leading US journal is a platform for the development of studies of interpersonal conduct and experience. There is an emphasis on empirical research (especially qualitative studies), but papers with a substantive focus on theory and conceptual development are also accepted.

The paper was accepted as relevant to the aims of the journal and sent out for peer review. The first correspondence from the editor (whose role in this instance was to aggregate peer reviewer comments and incorporate this with a personal response), held that the submitted draft of the paper had interest, showed promise and was 'intriguing although not entirely successful at this point'. The paper was praised for locating itself in the relevant literature and for demonstrating an excellent grasp of the realities of nursing. It was felt that, potentially, the paper could make a considerable contribution to this field. Allen was therefore encouraged to further revise and resubmit the manuscript, taking into account peer review comments.

Whilst positive about the potential contribution of the paper, all three reviewers uniformly focused on the 'boundary' theme and the links between this concept and the data presented (numbers refer to the individual peer reviewers):

> I am afraid I came away from this paper without having my understanding [of boundary work] deepened very much.
>
> (218)

> I do not see this paper as boundary work or at least not as how Gieryn saw it.
>
> (219)

> ... the paper never coheres into a compelling analysis of 'boundary work' ... the various extracts have an illustrative quality that is nicely descriptive, but they fail to build up to any concerted argument.
>
> (176)

Each reviewer provided instructions on what they thought needed to be changed, so the author could then take the necessary steps to alter content. Recommended reading was suggested, alongside specific actions regarding further exploration of the data and analysis:

> ... I think this paper/analysis needs to put more meat on the bones of its primary thesis ... I think it would be of use to include, at this point, a more developed discussion of this concept [boundary work], and then use this discussion to guide and illuminate the subsequent analysis.
>
> (218)

In Extract 4, for example, *why* is it funny for Dawn to say 'should we be doing that for doctors as well?' What if the same thing were said by nurses about a *subordinate* health care worker? … Wouldn't it be sociologically interesting to contrast the stories that nurses tell about doctors with those they tell about health care assistants? … Such an addition to the analysis would, I believe, get the manuscript beyond the rather well-understood conclusion that nurses 'accomplish shared perspectives' by telling us tales about how doctors sometimes are.

(219)

At the beginning and the end of the manuscript, the author offers three goals for the paper. It would help the reader if the individual analyses of data extracts were more explicitly linked to one (or more) of these goals. The author attempts to construct such linkages 'after the fact' in the 'Discussion' section, but for me it was 'too little, too late' … Perhaps more stated guideposts along the way would assist readers like me who need a little help in this regard.

(176)

On receipt of the reviewers' comments, the task of the author is to address the necessary revisions. Referees' opinions are rarely completely unanimous, and if the Editor does not give any clear guidance on revising the paper, the author is left to make an informed judgement about how best to respond. This will be influenced by their knowledge of the field, their dissemination plans, i.e. what it is they hoped to communicate to the research community, and how far any recommended changes can be accommodated whilst retaining fidelity to the paper's intellectual origins. It is important that referees' comments are considered in the round. This may result in some recommendations being rejected; as in responding to one set of comments others are rendered irrelevant. It may even lead to an author withdrawing a paper from the journal and seeking an alternative outlet for the work. Where there is confusion or conflict over comments, it can be helpful to contact the journal.

In this particular case, the sum of the reviewers' comments was more useful to the author than their individual contributions (Allen, personal communication). The revision of the paper did not entail attending slavishly to every single concern raised by the referees. Instead the reviewers' comments were considered together carefully in order to diagnose why the paper was not working at this stage. In the event, the paper was substantially revised. The most significant change was a narrowing of the study's focus, since the reviewers' comments indicated that the author had tried to attend to too many issues and, as a consequence, the over-arching boundary work focus was obscured.

With the comments addressed the revised manuscript was seen as being stronger, leaving reviewers 218 and 219 happy with the changes made.

> I have completed my review of the revised manuscript and find it a vastly improved paper ... I find the improvement of the paper be a positive testimony to the peer review process.
>
> (218)

> The revisions to this manuscript have been substantial – and more importantly effective. To my mind the author has rescued and turned it into a creative, interesting and important contribution to the literature on the practice of cultural/professional boundaries.
>
> (219)

This was not the end of the process; with reviewer 176 having reservations, implying that the narrative still did not offer a compelling account of boundary work. A more detailed discussion began around apparent philosophical contradictions in the manuscript, dealt with through a clear exchange of opinion. After several minor modifications the paper finally got accepted for publication, although reviewer 176's opinion stayed unchanged.

> While I appreciate all the hard and thoughtful work, I'm still not persuaded by the paper and its 'boundary work' argument ... from these data I do not share the author's view of the phenomenon ... in the broadest outline, it is certainly about symbolic interaction, and that's enough for me.
>
> (176)

This case study illustrates the positive side of the peer review process. Unlike case study 1, there was little doubt that the nature of the paper fitted the aims of the journal and it was therefore appropriately placed. The reviewers initially viewed the paper as flawed but with promise. There was subsequent transparent and detailed discussion, resulting in the production of a manuscript which would contribute intellectually to a particular community. That one reviewer did not see eye-to-eye with the author on several points should not be seen as negative. Such discussion is vital for the development of rigorous work. The same principle can be applied to statistical papers, where reviewers might question a potential flaw in the study design e.g. the sample size of the population under study. This should then prompt a dialogue between author and reviewer about the strength of the claims made from such data, resulting in the suggestion of possible changes and the production of a stronger paper to inform the reader.

Case studies 1 and 2 have drawn attention to one essential part of the dissemination process, that of relationship between author and output. Only by producing work of high quality in the appropriate medium can the next stage, i.e. interpretation of work, be carried out with any degree of success. Case study 3 throws some light on this link in the dissemination chain.

Case study 3: Relationship between published work and reader

In the first two case studies we have seen some research evaluators in action. This case study demonstrates how nurses acting in this capacity and also as users of research, can influence the dissemination of research findings, sometimes in a surprising way. It draws on Church and Lyne (1994) and Church (1992).

The story began when a midwife, attending a research preparatory course, was looking for a topic on which to base a formal literature review. She had recently become aware of a managerial decision to withdraw ring cushions from the midwifery unit, where they had been in use for many years to relieve perineal discomfort following vaginal delivery. When she enquired why this had been done, the answer was that research had shown that they caused thromboses and pressure sores. However, she realized that, in several years of practice, she had never seen a new mother with a pressure sore, and apparently neither had any of her colleagues. She therefore decided that an investigation of the research evidence would be an ideal topic for her review. She found that, over many years, the literature had clearly demonstrated a link between sustained intersurface pressure and both pressure damage and vascular compression leading to increased risk of thrombosis. Elderly, immobile and chronically ill people were considered to be at particular risk from the effects of increased pressure between their tissues and the substrate. However, there was no consensus about the strength or duration of pressure required to produce these effects and very little data concerning their effects in healthy people. There were frequent references in the nursing literature to the work of Lowthian (1985), stating that he had shown the circulation to be affected by the pressure exerted by ring cushions. Walsh and Ford (1998) interpret his writings to mean that he has *shown* that the pressure produced by a ring cushion *causes* circulatory impairment and *predisposes* to tissue breakdown.

Following the trail back to the 1985 paper, the midwife found that this reported a study of the intersurface pressures between the skull of a patient and an occipital ring cushion. Lowthian extrapolates from his observation of pressures and weights to the condition of the seated patient, calculating that this will produce intersurface pressures of about 35 mm Hg, which is above the level of arterial capillary pressure (32 mm Hg) in the nail bed of the healthy subject (Landis, 1930). Pressure of this order was accepted, at the time of this case study, as the threshold for the production of tissue injury (Carlson and King, 1990). He concludes that tissues *may* be damaged but does not produce any direct evidence that they are.

Through a succession of readers, Lowthian's original tentative conclusion, derived from work with immobilized patents, has been elevated to factual status, relating to newly delivered mothers (who are, in the main, healthy, mobile and very unlikely to remain seated for prolonged periods) through subtle shifts in the wording. The weight of the conclusion has shifted from 'may cause tissue breakdown', through 'predisposes to tissue breakdown' to 'causes pressure sores'. The effect was to remove from practice simple devices that, according to Grant and Sleep (1989), have been helpful to post partum mothers, enabling them to sit comfortably to feed their babies.

Shifting conclusions

The facts presented here refer to the time at which the literature review took place and do not take into account any subsequently produced evidence or guidelines. They are described in order to illustrate how the conclusion of a published work (or indeed, of any form of disseminated material) can be interpreted by successive readers. Minor semantic shifts can turn a tentative suggestion into a firmly held belief which impacts on education, management and practice.

This demonstrates the vulnerability of the tentative (some might say vague) conclusion to this type of distortion. The word 'may' has always been far too common in nursing writings, representing a reluctance to make a definitive statement that is not backed up by extensive references, something that appears to be ingrained in the education of nurses. It does have a proper place, when a categorical statement is not justified, but frequently it is used to cover a lack of intellectual rigour in published papers. What does it actually mean in this context? In linguistic terms 'may' is a modal verb, one which is associated with an obligation and is capable of more than one interpretation. It could mean, 'I do not know; the evidence, such as it is, is finely balanced. This is possibly the case or possibly not.' Alternatively: 'The weight of evidence inclines me to the belief that this probably is the case, but I cannot be certain' or even 'There is absolutely no evidence but my gut feeling leads me to think that this is the case.' In a more archaic sense it could also mean, 'This is permitted to be the case', a usage which often causes confusion to people learning English as a second language. The point is that this term has the potential to create ambiguity and leaves a vacuum in which all sorts of meanings can be generated.

Research of a more scholarly and less applied nature does, in fact, often have this as its very purpose. It is intended that a dialogue between reader and text should occur in this space (Traynor, 1999) and so words which suggest possibilities have a proper place here. We would argue that this issue is of more than semantic importance. It really matters in nursing research that the reader of published work should understand in what sense the authors are using words such as this, since subsequent use of the findings, including their interpretation to form part of the evidence base, will be affected by that understanding.

Given the eclectic nature of nursing research, its current situation and the variety of studies which it encompasses it is, in our opinion, most unlikely that nursing research reports will ever become as standardized as, for example, laboratory-based studies. This is probably all to the good, but it poses challenges for all involved in the dissemination of research. In this chapter we have glimpsed some of the ways in which the link between writer and reader can be influenced by extraneous forces, sometimes to change the message, sometimes to improve and move forward the thinking and sometimes to halt the process or distort the conclusion. Many people contribute to this chain of events, either directly or indirectly, and we suggest that all have a part to play in enhancing its effectiveness. Their contribution here is one aspect of their particular mode of engagement with research.

The research teacher clearly assists the research producer to develop competence, but a somewhat neglected part of this role is to inculcate the ability to write lucidly and argue logically. This is the foundation upon which the successful and accurate dissemination of research findings depends and unfortunately, for whatever reason, it is often an area of difficulty for nurse researchers. Positive steps can be taken within undergraduate or research preparatory programmes to remedy any deficits in previous educational experience, just as Keith Weeks has shown us in the case of mathematical skills. The research supervisor continues this process at undergraduate or postgraduate level and the research leader should be concerned to develop the writing skills of the whole team, as well as helping individuals and groups to prepare their publication strategies. This is a process needing dedicated time and purposeful activity.

The research manager has to be assured that project teams contain the required level of competence in report writing, or to take steps to develop individuals as part of the project costs. Failure to ensure this level of capability can affect the way that project outcomes are disseminated. Research producers are, of course, usually the people who write the reports for publication. It is their ultimate responsibility to produce such reports in the clearest possible language in order to convey their meaning to the desired audience. When the research is being planned, the research producers need to bear in mind the importance of having something to say when they have finished, or, in other words, to be able to tell the users something definite. This means designing the research so that it will yield an answer to some important question and expressing that answer with a degree of precision, even if this produces a report that is not very accessible to the general reader. As long as a report of this nature exists and is in the public domain, the research evaluators can access it and do the work of determining what it really means for the users with whom they work (who may, of course, also wish to appraise it in the same way if their role demands that they do and they posses the appropriate skills).

Research evaluators, working as reviewers and editors, exert a major influence on the whole process, as we have seen in this chapter. At its best, this can be a very positive influence. By challenging and stretching the author the quality of the paper can be improved.

Conclusion

In practical terms, the case studies considered in this chapter raise a number of important learning points for those new to nursing research and beginning to disseminate their work.

The purpose of dissemination

Be very clear about the purpose of your study and the reason for wishing to disseminate the findings. It is important to decide on the audience and to link purpose and audience to the selection of dissemination mode.

Choose the correct outlet for the work

If publication in a journal best fits this purpose, take time to understand the aims and scope of each journal you consider, perhaps discussing this with someone who has already published in that journal or even writing to the editor to seek clarification.

Engagement with the review process

Think about how you will respond to the editor's initial reaction. Prepare for, and do not be discouraged by, a less than enthusiastic response. If you really want the paper to appear in that journal, it is essential to take the editor's advice. Such decisions may need to be balanced with your sense of the intellectual fidelity to the original study. Persevere when you receive the reviewers' comments, even if you feel that they are living on another planet. Maybe share the comments with a colleague who is not involved in the work, to provide an impartial view and help to use them constructively. Recognize that the review process, properly used, has the potential to take the work forward and improve its presentation to the desired audience.

References

Allen, D. (2001) 'Narrating nursing jurisdiction: atrocity stories and boundary-work', *Symbolic Interaction*, 24, 1–28.

Amin, M. and Mabe, M. (2000) 'Impact factors: use and abuse', *Perspectives in Publishing*, 1, 1–6.

Banyard, L.V. and Miller, K.L. (1998) 'The powerful potential of qualitative research for community psychology', *American Journal of Community Psychology*, 26, 485–505.

Bishop, V. (2004) 'Knocking down ivory towers: publish and be damned', in V. Bishop and D. Freshwater (eds) *Nursing Research in Context: Appreciation, Application and Professional Development*, Basingstoke, Palgrave.

Blackburn, C., Graham, H. and Scullion, P. (1997) 'Disseminating research findings on women's smoking to health practitioners: Findings from an evaluation study', *Health Education Journal*, 56, 113–24.

Bond, S. (2002) *UOA10 – Nursing. Overall Assessment of the Sector*, London: HERO.

Carlson, C.E. and King, R. (1990) 'Prevention of pressure sores', *Annual Review of Nursing Research*, 8, 35–56.

Carter, D. (1996) 'Barriers to the implementation of research findings in practice', *Nurse Researcher*, 4, 30–40.

Church, S. (1992) 'The case of the disappearing doughnut', Unpublished thesis, Sheffield City Polytechnic.

Church, S. and Lyne, P.A. (1994) 'Research-based practice: some problems illustrated by the discussion of evidence concerning the use of a pressure relieving device in nursing and midwifery', *Journal of Advanced Nursing*, 19, 513–18.

Cronenwett, L.R. (1995) 'Effective methods for disseminating research findings to nurses in practice', *Nursing Clinics of North America*, 30, 429–38.

Dixon-Woods, M., Fitzpatrick, R. and Roberts, K. (2001) 'Including qualitative research in systematic reviews: Opportunities and problems', *Journal of Evaluation and Clinical Practice*, 7, 125–33.

Emden, C. (1996) 'Manuscript reviewing: too long a concealed form of scholarship?', *Nursing Inquiry*, 3, 195–9.

Grant, A. and Sleep, J. (1989) 'Perineal care', in I. Chalmers, M. Enkin and M. Keirse (eds) *Effective Care in Pregnancy and Childbirth*, Oxford: Oxford University Press.

Holt, J., Barret, C., Clarke, D. and Monks, R. (2000) 'The globalization of nursing knowledge', *Nurse Education Today*, 20, 426–31.

Landis, E.M. (1930) 'Micro-injection studies of capillary blood pressure in human skin', *Heart*, 15, 209–28.

Lomas, J. and Haynes, R.B. (1987) 'A taxonomy and critical review of tested strategies for the application of clinical practice recommendations: from "official" to "individual" clinical policy', *American Journal of Preventative Medicine* 4, 77–94.

Lowthian, P. (1985) 'A sore point', *Nursing Mirror*, 161, 30–2.

Lyne, P., Allen, D., Satherley, P. and Martinsen, C. (2002) 'Improving the evidence base for practice: a realistic method for appraising evaluations', *Journal of Clinical Effectiveness in Nursing*, 6, 81–8.

McDonnell, A., Davies, S., Brown, J. and Shewan, J. (1997) *A Detailed Investigation of the Implementation of Research Based Knowledge by Practice Nurses in Relation to Cardiovascular Disease and Stroke Prevention*. Final report to the NHS Research and Development Executive. Sheffield: University of Sheffield.

Murphy, E., Dingwall, R., Greatbatch, D., Parker, S. and Watson, P. (1998) 'Qualitative research methods in health technology assessment: a review of the literature', *Health Technology Assessment*, London: Health Technology Assessment.

Newell, R. (2000) 'Writing academic papers: the clinical effectiveness in nursing experience', *Clinical Effectiveness in Nursing*, 4, 93–8.

NHS (1996) 'Information needs assessment report', London: NHS Executive.

Popay, J., Rogers, A. and Williams, G. (1998) 'Rationale and standards for the systematic review of qualitative literature in health services research', *Qualitative Health Research*, 8, 341–51.

Rafferty, A.M., Bond, S. and Traynor, M. (2000) 'Does nursing, midwifery and health visiting need a research council?', *Nursing Times Research*, 5, 325–35.

Rycroft-Malone, J., Harvey, G., Seers, K., Kitson, A., McCormack, B. and Titchen, A. (2004) 'An exploration of the factors that influence the implementation of evidence into practice', *Journal of Clinical Nursing*, 13, 913–24.

Sackett, D.L., Rosenberg, W., Gray, M.C., Muir, J.A., Haynes R., Richardson, B. and Scott, W. (1996) 'Evidence based medicine: what it is and what it isn't', *British Medical Journal*, 312, 71–2.

Scullion, P. (2002) 'Effective dissemination strategies', *Nurse Researcher*, 10, 65–77.

Thorne, S., Jensen, L., Kearney, M.H., Noblit, G. and Sandelowski M. (2004) 'Qualitative metasynthesis: reflections on methodological orientation and ideological agenda', *Qualitative Health Research*, 14, 1342–65.

Traynor, M. (1999) 'The problem of dissemination: evidence and ideology', *Nursing Inquiry*, 6, 187–97.

Van Teijlingen, E. and Hundley, V. (2002) 'Getting your paper to the right journal: a case study of an academic paper', *Journal of Advanced Nursing*, 37, 506–11.

Van Teijlingen, E., Rebbie, A.M., Hundley, V. and Graham, W. (2001) 'The importance of conducting and reporting pilot studies: the example of Scottish Births Survey', *Journal of Advanced Nursing*, 34, 289–95.

Van Weel, C. (2003) 'Translating research into practice – a three-paper series', *The Lancet*, 362, 1170.

Waddell, C. (2002) 'So much research evidence, so little dissemination and uptake: mixing the useful with the pleasing', *Evidence Based Nursing*, 5, 38–40.

Wakley, T. (1823) The Lancet – Preface, *The Lancet*, 1, 1–2.

Walsh, D. and Downe, S. (2005) 'Meta-synthesis method for qualitative research: a literature review', *Journal of Advanced Nursing*, 50, 204–11.

Walsh, M. and Ford, P. (1998) *Nursing Rituals: Research and Rational Actions*, Oxford: Heinemann Nursing.

Conclusion

Davina Allen and Patricia Lyne

The case studies analysed in Part II have provided a rich resource from which to consider the realities of nursing research. Some of the issues and learning points which have arisen are common to research in other fields, but many of them, overlaid as they are with the peculiar context in which nursing research is situated, have characteristics that are unique to the discipline. For each chapter in Part II we have identified the specific learning points that emerged from an analysis of nurses' engagement with different elements of the research process. In editing this book we tried to ensure that each of the case study chapters retained a focus on a particular aspect of the research process, yet as the case studies unfolded it was clear that there were many issues which were common to our contributors' stories. In this final chapter we attempt to draw the threads of our thinking together by reflecting on the broader insights for the research process that have emerged from the book as a whole.

In Chapter 6 we have revealed the many factors which influence the selection of a topic and how the interaction of service and professional agenda makes this a more complex undertaking in nursing than is the case in other disciplines. The time and skills necessary to this process are, in our view, often under-estimated and the action-oriented culture which characterizes nursing work can sometimes make it difficult to make the case for time to think. Rather like talking to patients, thinking is not always considered as real work. We have identified strategies which can be deployed to make this process more manageable, and in particular have highlighted the importance of good supervision and the identification and involvement of key stakeholders at an early stage. In fact selecting a research topic in the nursing context is frequently much more than a matter for the research producer alone. Research supervisors and research leaders have a role in assisting the research producer to strike a balance between passion for the subject and what is realistic and feasible, given all the competing influences in play.

Having settled upon a topic for study, the next step in the process usually entails the development and negotiation of a proposal through key gate-keeping committees. In Chapter 7 we argued that gatekeepers, such as funding bodies and ethical committees, replicate many of the power imbalances seen in the practice arena, and are strongly influenced by dominant medical and management discourses. We have shown how their deliberations take place in a context where there is lack of clarity over some procedural matters and debates concerning the characteristics of research (as opposed to audit or service improvement). This creates an important role for the research leader in ensuring that gatekeeper agenda are well-understood, that sufficient time is allowed for all the activities necessary to satisfy their demands and that research producers are encouraged to persevere and challenge constructively.

Chapters 8, 9, and 10 in different ways considered nurse researchers' engagement with processes of data generation. They point to how professional and practitioner identities can be both a resource and a liability in this context. We have seen that practical engagement with a field can be central to shaping the emerging research focus, and how professional status and understanding can be vital to securing research access. It is important for nurse researchers to value this insider knowledge, whilst recognizing its attendant dangers. A clear message to emerge from these chapters is the need for reflexivity in the research process and the adoption of appropriate theoretical frameworks in order to safeguard against bias or limited vision through an over-familiarity with the field. Helping to achieve this balance is an important role for research supervisors.

For nurses researching their own clients, the case studies in Chapter 10 reveal the impact of medical discourses in relation to research of this kind and highlight the need for absolute clarity of purpose at all stages of the research, so that methodological choices can be justified. Chapters 6 and 9 also highlight some of the tensions that can arise for those who adopt a dual nurse/researcher role in mediating the diverse social worlds of academe and practice and their divergent cultures and associated frameworks for action. We also point to the particular challenges faced when research takes place in one's own organization and the role of colleagues as research influencers in shaping the progress of the research. These issues need to be properly understood by research leaders, managers and supervisors.

In Chapter 11 we reflected on our own intellectual biographies in order to demonstrate how the intersection of different frameworks of understanding with individual trajectories produces a range of unique sets of skills and predispositions within the nursing research community, which is particularly relevant to the analysis and interpretation of data. This could be a strength if properly managed within a research team or group. An important role for research leaders and managers is to foster and capitalize on the intellectual heritage of team members and to enable specific additional (perhaps subject specific) expertise to be added where needed. It is also important for this diversity of approach to be recognized in order to ensure that neophyte researchers are appropriately matched with supervisors.

In Chapter 12 we considered the role of nurses in multidisciplinary research teams, which are increasingly becoming a necessity in securing external research funding. Our case studies have illustrated that multidisciplinary research requires that individuals with diverse professional agenda and intellectual biographies work together with the potential for conflict. It is important for research leaders and managers to allow time for the development of shared understanding amongst team members. For nurse researchers these challenges are compounded by the expectation that power imbalances that characterize the service setting will be replicated in the research context. It is essential, therefore, that nurse researchers are clear about their mode of engagement in multidisciplinary research teams and the nature of their particular contribution to the research endeavour.

Finally in Chapter 13, we focused on the process of disseminating research findings. Relatively little has been written on this topic in the nursing research context. The case studies in this chapter highlight that the singular characteristics of nursing research can result in the production of non-standard research outputs which can make dissemination challenging at times. The importance of clearly identifying the target audience for the work is identified which, in some instances, may require different versions of a paper to be produced for academic and practitioner readership. The case studies highlight the importance of perseverance and the value of constructive engagement with the peer review process.

In writing this book we had three inter-related aims: to 'tell it as it is' in order to share those experiences that often remain hidden from view in standard research texts, to provide a critical analysis of the nursing research context and to bring these two threads together in the form of practical advice to those embarking on the research journey for the first time. For this reason we have tended to focus on the challenges faced by those who work in the field. In so doing we hope we have not painted too depressing a picture. Other themes which emerge from the studies described here and from the process of editing this manuscript include the passion the authors express for their subjects, the personal growth engendered by the research process and the emotions that such intense engagement with a field of interest can evoke. Whilst we have argued strongly for recognition of research as a specialist skill, we have also highlighted the different kinds of knowledge that can be brought to the research process, of which clinical experience is a vital ingredient. Nursing's lack of research capacity should not be allowed to over-shadow how members can contribute to research in this respect. On a more personal note, we have both found research to be an endlessly rewarding activity. Patricia, now planning to retire from an academic role, would do it all over again (perhaps using this text to avoid learning some painful lessons). She considers that the present day would be a good time to be embarking on a research career in nursing since, despite all the challenges we have described, research in the profession seems poised at last to achieve its potential by identifying and valuing the variety of ways in which we engage with research. Davina, relatively recently appointed to a senior research leadership role, also looks to the future with optimism and the opportunities this presents for her continuing intellectual development through participation in the progression of policies and strategies to promote nursing research, personal scholarship and the support of others embarking on this journey.

Index

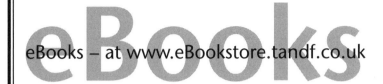